This

ABC of Change for Doctors

Susan E Kersley MB BCh MEd BA

Foreword by
David Haslam

Radcliffe Publishing
Oxford • Seattle

Radcliffe Publishing Ltd
18 Marcham Road
Abingdon
Oxon OX14 1AA
United Kingdom

www.radcliffe-oxford.com
Electronic catalogue and worldwide online ordering facility.

British Library Cataloguing in Publication Data

A catalogue record for this book is available from the British Library.

ISBN-10 1 85775 762 9
ISBN-13 978 1 85775 762 0

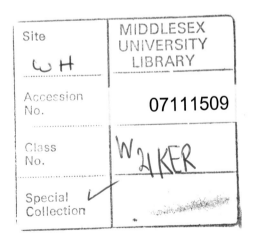
Typeset by Aarontype Ltd, Easton, Bristol
Printed and bound by TJ International Ltd, Padstow, Cornwall

To everyone who wants their life to be different;
It's as easy as ABC to change your life!

If you can imagine it, you can achieve it.
If you can dream it, you can become it.
William Arthur Ward

Contents

Foreword

There's nothing special about doctors. If you cut us, do we not bleed? We are just human beings, like everyone else on the planet. But all too often we don't behave as if this were true.

Few other professionals have to deal with the traumatic, upsetting, and distressing problems that affect their fellow humans in the same way that we do. When others face these problems they are likely to get support, an opportunity to unload, and even counselling. Doctors don't. Doctors often feel trapped by their altruism, unable to express how hurt they feel, how difficult they find the work, how unhappy they are with their lives.

It doesn't have to be this way. I remember when I first started to work in my practice, I realised that I was likely to work in that self same room longer than I had lived — and so it has worked out. But if you keep on doing what you always did, you'll keep on getting what you always got.

And change is the key to our sanity. Whilst it is all too easy to feel sucked into a downward spiral, feeling yourself to be a powerless victim in the never ending cycle of NHS and societal change, this will be a recipe for an unfulfilled and damaged life.

Susan Kersley's beautifully straightforward and logical book shows any doctor how to take back the control. You may not be able to change the NHS, but you can change your life. I'm all too aware that this sentence sounds much like the worst form of psychobabble, but the simple fact is that it really is true. Even the simplest of steps can make a difference. A few years ago I realised that I started almost every day in a negative frame of mind. As a natural optimist this puzzled me. And then I realised that listening to the Today programme on Radio Four with its constant undertone of haranguing cynicism was not the best recipe for contentment. Switching to Radio Five — the same news, many more laughs, and too much football made a real difference.

A ridiculous example? Maybe. But taking such tiny steps, analysing what is wrong with your life, taking control rather than persisting in habitual behaviour, seeking advice, owning up to the fact that you — the person, the human, and not the doctor — really do matter, can make a remarkable difference to how you face today and the rest of your life.

I am delighted that Susan Kersley has written this book which can help you make the changes you currently only dream of. As the old cliché goes, life isn't a dress rehearsal. You're on the real stage. Act now.

David Haslam CBE
General Practitioner, Cambridgeshire
National Clinical Adviser to the Healthcare Commission
Former Chairman of Council of the RCGP
September 2005

About the author

Susan E Kersley was a medical practitioner for over 30 years. In 1997 she changed her life and became a life coach, writer and NLP (neurolinguistic programming) Practitioner. She coaches doctors on the telephone, wherever they live, and facilitates workshops to enable doctors to have a life.

Her first book, *Prescription for Change*, was published in 2003 by Runnelstone Books. The second edition was published in 2005 by Radcliffe Publishing. *The ABC of Change for Doctors* is her second book.

She is married to an orthopaedic surgeon, has three grown up children and lives in Cornwall, UK. Her website is www.thedoctorscoach.co.uk.

Acknowledgements

This book evolved from a series of articles called 'The ABC of Change' which originally appeared in the *British Medical Journal* during 2004. A huge thank you to Rhona MacDonald, former editor of *BMJ Career Focus*, for her incredible support and encouragement. Thanks also to the readers of the articles who encouraged me with their positive comments.

Thank you to my coaching clients who keep me informed of the present state of medical life, and to workshop participants who are willing to discuss and look at their lives differently.

As always, thanks to my husband Jonathan for his continuing love and support for my writing adventures.

Why an ABC?

This book offers you an ABC for change. You can read it from A to Z or open it at random when you have a spare minute or two. And that's the first challenge – to find the time to have a life. Medicine can engulf you. It doesn't have to. You can be a doctor and have a life too. Are you ready to find out ways to be a doctor and change the balance of your life? It could be as easy as ABC!

> *Creating an ABC liberates us from classifying things as rare or beautiful to demonstrate what we care about in the everyday. It is useful in that it levels everything, it reshuffles things and juxtaposes them in ways that surprise and make you think. This can change what we see, disperse our complacency, make things we take for granted seem new to us and encourage us to take action.*
>
> www.commonground.org.uk

> *Human beings, by changing the inner attitudes of their minds, can change the outer aspects of their lives.*
>
> William James

Making a major change in your life may take you on a 'Hero's Journey,' (an archetypal, mythical journey, described by Joseph Campbell[1]), with recognisable stages. When you think about the major changes you've made already in your life you may recognise the features. At every stage of the journey there is always the choice to continue, stay put or go back.

The journey begins with 'the call', the feeling inside you that things can't go on as they are, that something has to change. If you decide to ignore the call, you may find it stays in you, like a chronic ache. However, if you answer it, then the journey towards your goal has begun. As you move forwards you will find some people who help and encourage you, while others will do whatever they can to dissuade you from the path you've chosen. Some people may try to dissuade you because they are jealous or genuinely believe you are doing the wrong thing.

Others may encourage you because they wish they too had your courage and admire what you are doing. At some stage you may find yourself confused, sure you chose the wrong path, and be plagued by self-doubt and questioning. You may feel as though you are in a wilderness or on a rough and stormy sea. It's all part of the process for change. However, if you hang on, you will eventually see a light at the end of the tunnel and reach your goal. When you do, you may feel a strong sense of being where you are meant to be, and that everything on the way was worth it.

And yet ... you may be surprised to find, when you reach the end of your journey, that you feel as though it is like a return almost to where you started. However, you and your life *will* be different, there will be similarities and connections with how things were before, but you will be happy and content instead of frustrated and overwhelmed.

When this happens, the journey will have been worthwhile.

Reference

1 Campbell J (2003) *The Hero's Journey: Joseph Campbell on his life and work*. New World Library, Novato, CA.

A is for

Accept	**Anger**
Achievable	**Answer**
Action	**Assertive**
Ambition	**Assumptions**

Sometimes you reach a point in your life when you decide something has to change. You know there must be another way to live. There must be another way to cope with life as a doctor, so that you can have the time and energy to enjoy other things too. The big question to ask yourself is: 'Are you ready to discover what can be changed and **accept** the things which cannot?'.

If you really want your life to be different you have to explore this distinction. It's easy to let your daily routines govern your life so much that you are no longer able to recognise there may be another way. Look around and notice which of your colleagues seems to be managing more efficiently than you. Notice who goes home on time and who stays late each day. Have you ever considered talking to them about how they get through their clinic faster than you or how they cope with the administration? Doing so might give you some clues about the way you, too, might be more efficient and balance your life and work more effectively. Then you would be more able to decide what you actually want in terms of changing your life for the better. Until you know what your desired outcome is, you'll find it difficult to decide how to achieve it.

When you've thought about what you want to do, the next step is to weigh up the pros and cons of all the various options for making it happen. If you say that what you would like is to finish your work in the hospital or surgery on time, and not take any home with you, then you might consider whether this is *really* what you want.

Perhaps you enjoy appearing busy when you are at home and like having an excuse not to do any domestic chores. Maybe you would be bored if you went home with an empty briefcase and wouldn't know how to occupy yourself during the evening.

On the other hand, if you know you would be able to enjoy hobbies once again or spend time with family and friends, without worrying about a pile of work, then set your goals and decide to do whatever is needed to reach them.

If you've been trying to change your life for some time already and, in spite of your decision and determination, nothing ever seems to change for you, then you need to look again at what you say you hope to do. Make your mind up if your goal is potentially **achievable** by you. If it isn't something you feel passionately about, then you may find it difficult to make it happen.

When you recognise that your own needs are as important as those of others, then, however much you wonder about the pros and cons, however much you wonder if this is the right or the wrong way to move forward, you won't know for sure until you take that big plunge into the pool of uncertainty. You won't know until you take some **action**.

However tiny that action, it almost doesn't matter. But doing something is a vital part of the process and the only way to find out how changing something enables you to change the bigger things too. It helps you realise how putting yourself and your own needs to the forefront is a way to become better at what you do.

Perhaps you are scared because you think your **ambition** is so immense, you couldn't possibly achieve it. If so, break your goal into much smaller parts. For example, if you want to change to another specialty and it seems too daunting, start by finding out if any of your current training would be allowed for this. Find out precisely what's involved in time, examinations and work experience. When you've decided what needs to be done, and what the big picture looks like, then decide how to make the steps smaller, and make your mind up to complete them. For example, if you want to write a best seller start with writing articles and step by step build these into a book.

You might be stuck because you still feel a lot of **anger** about your life and the way it is, blaming the people who encouraged you to do what now you believe you didn't really want to do. If you became a doctor because you wanted to please an encouraging science teacher at school, or you grew up with the message 'everyone in your family does medicine, and so must you', or you wanted to help people and hadn't realised what a hard slog it would be and how tired you would get after a night on call, then you need to let go of that frustration. If you think you went into your particular branch of medicine or specialty because you liked the consultant and didn't want to upset her, then take a step back and re-think your priorities.

What do you want for your life? It's very important for you to forgive, in order to move onwards. Remind yourself how most people do what they consider is best for their children, friends, relatives or colleagues. However, people did what they did for you because of how they viewed their world, at the time, and were strongly influenced by their own experiences of life. You can't change the past but you can reassess it. Say to yourself 'That was then, and this is now', and be ready to move on and make the changes you want to make.

Changes happen, point by point. Your initial action might involve a conversation or an email with someone who has done what you want to do. Don't dismiss this initial research and investigation. Don't try to predict the **answer** you might get. People are usually very flattered when you ask them about something on which they are an expert. Do you see, already, in your mind's eye, how someone might respond? Can you imagine what they might say to you? Are you predicting how you might feel about their reaction? Are you, therefore, not doing something because of how you *imagine* that person would react to you?

Be clear what you want from them. You might tell them you've noticed they get through their work on time each day and that what you'd like is for them to give you some hints on how to do this too. Ask yourself what might happen if they became angry or upset? Visualise for a moment what might be the worst result of your request? And if it happened what might be the worst thing after that?

Preparation can be the key to successful interaction. Recognise that your fear is real and many people feel similarly at the thought of doing something different from their usual routine. Could you take a risk in order to affect the system in a small way and so make a difference to your life? Will you commit to taking a step out of your comfort zone today? To do this, centre yourself so you can deal with an adverse reaction. Think of your centre as the place below your umbilicus and take a breath into that place. Be like a tree, solid yet flexible, and you will be able to deal with all sorts of things.

You need to be **assertive** so that you recognise you have a right to be you and live the life you desire. This involves sticking to your question and using the 'stuck record' technique. Say whatever you want to say and just keep saying the same thing over and over in reply to whatever the other person says. If on the other hand you want to answer a request made of you, by saying 'no', don't give too many excuses, which may let the other person come back with counter reasons why you can fulfil their request,

Let go of your **assumptions** about your life, yourself, what you believe, and get the balance you want into your life. When you do this remember that being you is as important as your roles in relation to work, family and community. Don't neglect yourself any longer. Discover who you really are and start to have a life.

B is for

Balance	**Better**
Begin	**Body**
Behaviour	**Bone of contention**
Beliefs	**Boundaries**

When you look around at the way you spend your days, do you believe your present life is seriously out of **balance**? Do you feel as though everything is skewed towards hard work, long hours and very little recognition that there is anything much else? Is your life all slog and no play?

If you feel overwhelmed and fed up with life and would dearly love to **begin** to make changes, then don't wait any longer. Perhaps something happened to a friend or a colleague, or you've noticed how they seem to have a better quality of life than you, and you have, as a result, seen your own lifestyle in a different light. Perhaps you've suddenly begun to feel trapped in a way of life which you would like to change but believe you are powerless to do anything about.

However, there are always ways to change by making small improvements to your self-care, or in the way you do your job so that you too can have a more balanced life. This can have a profound effect not only on you but eventually on those around you too. When you make a decision to change something, you have to act differently in some way in order to have a new outcome, and when your routine changes others respond to you in a different way.

You can start by changing the way you think about yourself and your life. As you consider what you would do if everything was perfect, you will begin to realise that you do have choices and thinking about these can lead you to taking action.

What you are going to do by taking action is to change your **behaviour** so, as a result, your life will be altered too. At first this may seem difficult to do because, like learning to drive, new habits take time to become automatic, and you have to consciously make sure that you do the new thing every day. You may have to place a tick on a list each day for at least the next three weeks for your new action to become routine. Remember what it was like when you first learned to drive a car. You had to think about everything, for example looking in the mirror, changing gear, using the clutch correctly. Now you may find you take a journey and reach your destination without consciously realising any of that. You may even have forgotten which way you went. Just like driving, the things which seem so difficult to you now can eventually become things you will do quite automatically.

However, in order to take the important first step, it is necessary to look at your inner **beliefs** and values. These are what fuel your actions day by day. They are what drives you, what life is all about for you, and what helps you experience the world the way you do. The trouble is, you may not even be aware of how much these influence your thought processes and actions every day. Your beliefs and values affect the way you see the world, and may have been the reason for you being stuck and explain why you make assumptions about what you can or can't do differently. You may have always assumed that certain things just 'are' and can never be changed. A useful skill to develop is to be able to differentiate between things which can never be changed and those which theoretically could be. Sometimes it takes someone else to point these out to you, because when you are deeply involved in a situation you may find it difficult to know that there could be a different way to do things.

Beliefs tend to be the 'shoulds' in your life and they become the rules you live by. It is a widespread belief among doctors that they should be able to deal with stress, they should put work above all else, even if this erodes unacceptably into their own time and space, and they should keep going even if they feel ill. Do you recognise these sorts of 'shoulds' in your life? 'Shoulds' have usually been ingrained in you since childhood and, even now, may be a huge influence on the way you behave. When you understand this and appreciate that you can change your beliefs, and as a result your behaviour too, then now might be the time to let go of those which no longer serve a purpose for you.

You can do this by considering how, instead of knowing you *should* do something, you might feel **better** when you realise you have a choice. You *could* do something, but only if you choose to do so. Knowing you have a choice is very empowering. Instead of 'I *should* take work home with me each evening', you could say 'I *could* take work home with me each evening, if I *choose* to do so'. Try it and notice the difference!

Notice too how you stand or sit. It's easy to revert back to a childlike posture when you think about your parents telling you what to do. If you want transformation, it helps to change not only your thoughts and actions but also your physical self. It helps to get into the **body** of an adult. As you tell yourself to do this you will notice a subtle straightening of the spine, a change of facial expression, a relaxation of the shoulders, and this may be all it takes to move you into the possibility of being different.

If you want to change your working conditions and you go along to your manager, your consultant or whoever you believe can influence these decisions and speak quietly, apologetically, in a childlike way, you may find that the response is different from when you walk in, knowing you have a reasonable request to make and you intend to discuss this in an adult and sensible way. Remind yourself that you are grown-up and, even though sometimes you might feel as if you are in the body of a child, you are more likely to reach a satisfactory outcome when you engage another person, adult to adult. Your interactions take place not only with what you say but also with how you are and how you regard yourself in the world.

The source and the long-term effects of your *shoulds* might be a **bone of contention** to you. You may feel angry when you think about how those beliefs have affected your life and your actions for so long. You might find it difficult to believe that you can challenge the ideas which have informed your behaviour for most of your life and still have such a powerful influence on your thoughts today. Think about these things from an emotionally neutral standpoint and ask yourself if they serve you today. You don't have to change everything. You will find that the majority of your values are still valid and valuable today. However, it will help to tease out those which are not.

It can be a useful exercise to look deeper at a belief you have to find out what it means to you. If you feel strongly that you must stay late each evening, what does this mean to you? Does it come from believing hard work and long hours are good? Is there a conflict between this belief and one which tells you family and friends are important? When you think about 'the big picture', what is the most important to you?

Everyone has their own personal **boundaries**. They are about what you are prepared to accept or put up with before you say 'sufficient' or 'stop'. Where do you draw the line around yourself? There is always a moment or a situation when you say 'that's it, no more'. When you become aware of them, boundaries can be changed and you can train yourself to stop sooner, if, for instance, long hours is your issue.

Perhaps you've become aware of how often you are asked to do something extra because people know you always say 'yes'. Have you noticed how they prefix the request by telling you no one else is available to do it, because they are all too busy, that all the others are too occupied, but not you? Or are they able to set boundaries better than you? There is a common expectation of colleagues that if you work part time, you have the extra time available to do more tasks, because if you are not at work that time is 'free'. This is another example of belittling your boundaries by the person making the request of you and of you thinking your own time is less important than work commitments.

What would you be saying 'yes' to, if you said 'no' more often? Can you begin to recognise how important it is to look after yourself more, and prioritise what you will do to live your life in a more balanced way? Become more aware and look after your own needs for a change. Ask yourself what would actually happen if you don't agree to do the next extra favour someone asks you to do? Who could do it? What happens if no one does? Is it truly your and only your responsibility? You may be agreeing to do something which could easily be done by someone else or not be done at all. How much more will you continue to tolerate before you say 'no' or 'enough is enough'?

Who defines your personal boundaries, *you* or *someone else*? Be more assertive. Let others know that 'As from next week I will no longer be able to do such and such'. At what point will you say 'I can't stand this anymore', and mean it? Too often you let others define where *their* boundaries are, and expect yours to be the same as theirs.

What is vital is to be clear about *your* personal boundaries. If, for example, one of yours is about stopping work to go home at a certain time, then be clear about what tasks you can leave until the following day. In this way you can maintain that boundary. If you think there is still too much to do, begin to look at your working day and consider how to be much more efficient. If you have to write notes about each patient and find it difficult to do as you go along, and as a result have a backlog at the end of the day, think about how you could reorganise your appointments in order to do this necessary task as you go through the day. You might find that building in a gap of a few minutes between patients' appointments would enable you to do this. If you are in a specialty in which you allow a long appointment time, perhaps you could revise this and set new boundaries. Don't forget to let those involved, the patients and the administration staff, know what you are doing so they co-operate and support you.

If interruptions while you are seeing patients slows you down, decide on a time each day when you don't mind queries and phone calls so that you can do the work with patients more efficiently. You *can* say 'no' to things which are not a priority and recognise what can be done by someone else, or not be done as often, or even at all. When you do this you will start to change — not only you, but others, too, in response to what you do.

C is for

Choice	**Compliment**
Clarity	**Conditions**
Coach	**Confidence**
Coaching	**Conversation**
Commitment	**Critic**

If you are fed up with the way life is for you and imagine there is nothing you can do about it because there is no alternative, then take a deep breath and be willing to consider something completely different. When you are thinking about a situation from your perspective of being there, it's difficult to realise that you always have a **choice**, even if you think you haven't. You can do something or not do something. You can say 'yes' or you can say 'no'.

To make changes, saying 'no' more often is a vital skill to develop because your overwhelm and stress may be largely due to doing too much. Since you are a compassionate person, and a member of a caring profession, you may find that saying 'no' to a request is one of the most difficult things to do. When people ask you to do something they expect you to agree to do it as their personal experience of you confirms this. They know that if everyone else is too busy you will agree because you always do and are too kind to refuse.

However, someone asking you to do something doesn't mean you have a commitment to do so. At the moment of the request you can decide whether to agree or refuse. You don't have to give more than a simple reason such as 'sorry I'm too busy today'. Beware of getting into a discussion about what you might be too busy doing. At this stage the other person may tell you how to deal with this or that, or, if you agree to the request, you may decide that seeing your friend is less important than dictating another letter.

Think about yourself and your own needs for a while and notice what happens when you reflect on what you believe about yourself and your needs and as a result how your behaviour changes. You may surprise your colleagues when you do or say something different and at first they may think you aren't serious. This is where your own determination and confidence has to be unambiguous not only to you but to others too.

To move forward you need some **clarity** about where you are going. Define, in as much detail as possible, your desired outcome. A useful technique is to ask yourself questions about your vision or goal beginning with Who? What? Why? When? and How?. It's not enough to know what you *don't* want any more. You have to be clear about what you *do* want.

If you find it a challenge to be specific then be sure about how you will know when you've achieved. If you say you want to enjoy your job, begin to define what 'enjoyment' of your job would mean to you. When you do this you will be more able to know when you've succeeded.

Deciding how to make your goal 'measurable', is part of having a SMART goal (a goal which is specific, measurable, achievable, realistic and timed). Is this something you can do on your own? It may be, but, on the other hand, it's very useful to have some support.

You may find it valuable to find someone, such as a **coach** or mentor to talk to about your plans. The advantage of this sort of encouragement is that the person you speak to is not attached to the outcome of your discussion and he or she may be able to give you an objective view of what you are doing. With **coaching**, a powerful process occurs. By discussion and challenging questions you begin to think differently about your situation. By being able to talk and be listened to, you are able to find ways to do what you want, even when you previously thought there were few or no options for change. You feel supported by a person who sustains and motivates you and yet has no agenda except for your own. The net result of this is your **commitment**, which becomes stronger and things start to happen. Because you make promises to do something different, something to move yourself towards your new situation, you feel accountable and that in itself is a powerful enabler for change.

Professional coaching is an ongoing partnership that helps clients produce fulfilling results in their personal and professional lives. Through the process of coaching, clients deepen their learning, improve their performance, and enhance their quality of life. During each meeting, with their coach, the client chooses the focus of conversation while the coach listens and contributes observations and questions. This interaction creates clarity and moves the client into action. Coaching accelerates the client's progress by providing greater focus and awareness of choice.
The International Coach Federation

You can talk to your coach about where you are today and where you want to be, rather than what went on in the past. Coaching facilitates you to focus on what you need to do to change and allows you to explore ways to do this by discussion of different options, ways to follow through, how to avoid potential barriers to change and how to deal with them if they happen.

At a conference entitled *Improving Working Lives for Doctors* (October 2003),[1] several speakers recognised doctors as people, not only as members of the medical profession, but as people entitled to address their personal needs as well as those of partners, families and communities. They confirmed how important it is to be content, happy and have a good work–life balance. For too long the culture of medicine has been about medical work taking precedence over all other aspects of life. These ideas apply just as much to other busy professionals too.

Part of having an outstanding work–life balance is a supportive network, which could include a coach or mentor to talk to on a regular basis. This would be very empowering and enable more doctors to balance their lives more effectively.

A coach is someone onto whom you can offload and bounce ideas, and receive unconditional positive support and encouragement at whatever stage you are at in your career or your life. Although suggested for times of transition, such as for new consultants or for 'doctors in difficulty', coaching can benefit all doctors. Perhaps, some doctors at the top of the profession, who are highly successful professionally but failures in their personal lives, find it difficult to talk about these personal things to friends and colleagues. If this applies to you, then you may discover the benefit of having someone at the end of the phone to talk to on a regular basis.

A coach is not only someone to talk to, but also someone who will **compliment** you on your achievements. That, in itself, is highly motivating. Among medics, there is too much of being told what you did wrong, whether you are a medical student or a junior doctor, and this can lead to the unfulfilled desire for perfection in many doctors. As a way to learn, there is much power in first being told you did something well before being criticised for doing something wrong.

Coaching results in an improvement in your work–life balance, especially when the **conditions** of your present life overwhelm you. You learn ways to communicate more effectively so that you can deal with colleagues and patients more effectively and improve your circumstances.

When you have a happy life, both at work and at home, you are more likely to have the **confidence** to be an effective and efficient professional. You will recognise the importance of having time away from work to recharge your batteries, enjoy the company of family and friends, to take part in community activities and to care for your own body, mind and soul.

Are you really clear about what is important for *you* in your life? Are you sure about what success means to *you?* So often you get swept along by someone else's definition in relation to the job to apply for, the research to be done, and the conferences to attend. Are all these things congruent with what is important to you? There is no right or wrong answer. You can do what you feel drawn towards rather than what someone else has told you that you *should* do.

Start a **conversation** with those people who are important to you. By talking and listening you can explore your ideas with another person. As you notice both your and their reactions you are better able to formulate your plans. Perhaps now you will be more aware of the way the person you talk to sees their world, and what is important to them. Remember, we all experience the world differently and the way you experience life is unlikely to be the same as the person telling you to apply for the job somewhere you don't want to go.

Recognise that life is for living now rather than in some theoretical time in the future. You can be successful and happy and enjoy other parts of your life as well as medicine. You may daydream of a better life and then let the vision be pushed away by an internal voice, your inner **critic**, which will find reasons to delay. There may also be people who try to dissuade you, even your friends and family or your colleagues, who can't understand what's got into you.

Listen, be aware, answer the justification why you mustn't do something with all the reasons why you must, then plan what you will do, sooner rather than later. It is important to consider the things which might go wrong so that you can decide how you would deal with the situation if the worst scenario happens. That's being realistic.

However, once you've considered the objections and ways to cope with them, make your plans and put them into action. If you believe we are all on this earth for a reason, then perhaps now is the time to find and start to fulfil your life purpose, whatever that may be.

Reference

1 http://www.dh.gov.uk/PolicyAndGuidance/HumanResourcesAndTraining/Model/Employer/ImprovingWorkingLives

D is for

Daily	**Demand**
Dare	**Do it**
Declaration	**Dream**
Delegate	**Dump**

When you are fed up it's easy to complain, find fault with everyone else and forget about yourself. There is a common assumption that being upset has nothing to do with you and is caused by something or someone else, and dealing with it by being confrontational will bring about change. Generally all it does is start an argument, with both sides becoming more entrenched and resistant to doing anything different.

When you don't like a situation, much of that feeling comes from the way you deal with it. If your train is cancelled you might be very annoyed because you'll be late for a meeting, or you could recognise that you will still arrive in time for the coffee break and the first talk didn't look very interesting anyway.

If you continue doing things in the same way, do you think anything will change? If you want something which is not happening now, then something has to alter. The only person who has the power to do this is you. It is no good telling yourself how you want the other person to behave differently because you are likely to be disappointed. You can only change yourself. You have to start by examining what you do in the situation, how you react to the circumstances and how you could behave differently. This might be as simple as doing something with a smile rather than a scowl. It might be doing the task as quickly as reasonably possible instead of worrying about it all day.

When you change yourself and the way you react, this may have a knock-on effect on the others and so the change you want in the other person or people may well happen. What you have to do may be to communicate more clearly about what you want or don't want. This involves listening more effectively, as well as being able to make a request clearly and without aggression or threat. So you have to start the transformation you want in others by changing yourself first.

If you don't know how to change yourself in the situation you are concerned about, or even what you want or how you want it, then you could begin by committing to the introduction of some new regular **daily** habits into your life such as eating five pieces of fruit or brushing your teeth more often, or other ways to improve the quality of your life. When you eat more healthily and take more exercise, perhaps walking some or all of the distance to work, you begin to feel better in yourself and are better able to decide how to change the big things.

Your new habits might be bits and pieces you would do anyway or you may decide to introduce new routines. These may be what you think you could do and really want to do, but don't get around to doing. This might be something such as joining a choir or clearing your email Inbox each day. Whatever it is, by allocating time to something which you've been procrastinating about, you will be improving your own self-care and making a difference to your life for the better too. It takes about three weeks to integrate a new habit so don't give up too soon!

Think of several things which would be fairly easy to do and make a promise to yourself, or preferably someone else as a witness, to do them. Your words lead to action. You might find it helps to make a chart and add a tick as you complete each task.

It's one thing to talk about how fed up and frustrated you are with your life but it takes courage to make a start. It takes some nerve to challenge the system. Everyone else seems to be coping, but are they really? You may notice your colleagues seem stressed too, or there may be some you know who are having 'time off' for stress-related illness. You may know some doctors who cope by drinking heavily or who self-medicate. Initiating change is a powerful thing to do. It can have a fantastic ripple effect.

So discover if you **dare** to be the one who will do this, the one who will challenge your normal routine and decide to do something different. When you retire would you rather regret what you haven't done or would you prefer to be proud that you were able to bring what you wanted into your life and, by default, into the lives of others too. Because when you change for a better life, you will inspire others to change their lives too.

However, it's not enough to say something such as, 'I don't want this to happen any more'. If you want change you have to make a **declaration**. This is a statement not only of the situation as it is but also of what you intend to do. 'I can't stand this any more and I have decided instead to do so and so in future . . .', or 'I'm not prepared to continue working at home each evening so I've decided to dictate my letters and write my notes after each patient appointment. Therefore, in future, I would like you to leave a 10-minute gap between appointments. This will give me the chance to do these tasks and also to catch up when a patient takes longer than expected.'

These words lead to action, by you, by the receptionist and by the patient. They will have a profound effect on your life, the life of your partner and your family, when you no longer work at home every evening and, as a result, you have more energy and enjoy life much more. The words give the listener and yourself the expectation about something which from now on will be different. The words do more than just stating an opinion. They are the precursor to action. Take a deep breath and state what you are going to do. Announce what you are going to do to yourself, to your notebook, to your friends and family and to your colleagues. You could even shout it from the top of a mountain if there is a convenient one nearby.

If, however, you are still frustrated by wanting to do more, you might find it useful to become more time-aware in order to discover how you actually spend your day. By logging your activities during the day, you may be surprised at how long you spend on the telephone or how many patients over-run their allotted time slot. When you recognise the areas in which you could improve your efficiency or gain insight into how you waste time, you will find it becomes easier to identify how to free up time to introduce new activities or priorities.

If, at the moment, your main concerns are dealing with the working day and getting everything done in a reasonable time, then, by knowing what you do and when you do it, you may find ways to do things more efficiently. Notice who copes well and find out what they do differently from you. There may be some useful things to learn. However busy you are, you may discover ways to be better organised in how you manage your work. This may mean a change for you, from a haphazard way of working to discovering or devising better systems and becoming more organised.

Could you devise procedures to automate, as much as possible, some of what you do? Notice your inefficiencies and decide to be more streamlined. If you are a bit of a control freak or a perfectionist, you may have to let go of your need to do everything yourself, and of the idea that only you can do a good job, to be more willing to **delegate** to someone else (especially if you teach them the skills needed to do the job efficiently and well). Tell and show them clearly what you want and by when.

What may seem obvious to you, may be a mystery to the other person, so give them lots of support and encouragement so that they learn to do the job as well as you. Then step back and trust them to do the job while you get on with something else. If you find delegation very difficult, then you are in good company. You know you do what has to be done in a way which seems right to you. When someone else does the same task they may approach it very differently. When you know what the piece of work has to achieve you might better be able to judge the person to delegate to, by the result you want rather than their process for achieving this. Some people want to know all the theory about something. Others prefer to watch someone doing the task so that they can copy the procedure. Neither approach is right or wrong, just different.

Some of what you **demand** of yourself and of others may be unrealistic and stressful for all concerned. You may learn something useful from the person you delegate to, perhaps about ways you could do jobs more quickly and effectively. What you try to cram into your day could probably be done more resourcefully, so the more you learn about better ways to achieve the same result, the easier you may find it is to just **do it** yourself quickly and successfully, rather than offloading onto others. If you can't work out how, look around at your colleagues who are managing something similar much more promptly than you. Have a chat with them about how they do it. Ask them to teach you the way.

How about planning for the future? Not everyone has clear plans for next week let alone a five-year plan. Don't worry if your **dream** of a new life seems somewhat hazy. As you start to think about your whole life in a more balanced way, and begin to understand there are ways you could be fulfilled apart from work, you will become clearer about what in your day-to-day routine needs to modified.

Organising your day more efficiently is a good way to begin. At the beginning of each day prioritise what has to be done and what can wait. Notice if better planning eliminates some of the stress of tasks which have a completion time. If you know you have to present a paper to a meeting don't leave the preparation to the last minute. Plan the time to think about what message you want to convey and the slides you will show, so there is plenty of time to plan the presentation.

Equally important as delegation and more efficiency is deciding what to stop doing completely. What could you **dump**? So many things, both at home and at work, become routine and no one really knows why, persisting because 'that's the way things have always been done round here'. Do you dictate your letters at the end of each clinic instead of after seeing each patient? Do you have departmental or practice meetings in the evening instead of during the working day? Small changes to routines such as these can have a profound and positive effect on the morale of not only you but also your colleagues too.

When you've decided what to pass on to someone else to do, accepted and let go of time wasters and been as efficient as you can be with what is left, you can use the time you've made available to do something you really want. Don't wait until the time is 'right', start with something today. Even clearing a drawer or throwing away some journals will start the process. Let the changes begin.

E is for

Easy	**Encouragement**
Elation	**Endure**
Emotion	**Entrepreneur**
Empathy	**Excitement**

When you fall into bed after a busy time on-call and you wish the phone or bleep had never been invented and could be silenced forever, it may be difficult to believe how, one day, you might look back at this time of overwhelm and indecision and wonder why you took so long to get around to doing what you wanted. As you consider the changes you would like to make, yet keep putting off the time to do something, you may expect the moment you step out of your comfort zone to be unbelievably difficult. However, when you eventually do it, you will find that the experience is something else. You will look back at how you felt before, and reflect at how the journey seemed unexpectedly **easy**, compared with how you imagined it would be.

During the process of change to transform your life there may be days when everything goes really well and other days when you feel like giving up completely. However, this is part of the process and if you keep your eye on the goal until you finally reach it, you will know, for sure, it was worth all the hazards on the way, to experience the **elation**, which comes when you achieve.

Do you remember how it felt to pass your medical degree, put your first drip up or handle your first delivery? At the time you may have been incredibly nervous and imagined you could never get anything right and yet somehow you learned what to do and with a good teacher to help, you managed, eventually, to know what to do. Yes, those emotions will happen again when something you've been dreaming about for ages actually takes place because you've taken the necessary actions.

It's an **emotion** which is difficult to describe. It may be a mixture of delight and sadness, a combination of feelings about your success in achieving and regret about what you've left behind. It may be amazement at what you've been able to accomplish when you set your mind to it, in spite of any real or perceived opposition. You may tend to undermine your potential and not realise how something which seemed so difficult may turn out to be much easier than expected.

Once you've experienced this joy you will be able to show **empathy** and encouragement to others who want to change their lives too. You can tell them how you managed, explain how you went ahead against all the odds, how your doubts held you back for a while and then how you bravely did what you did. Doing this will motivate others to do what they want to do and their changes will, in turn, inspire you too. You will realise you are not in isolation but that every action has a reaction in others. The ripples spread outward a long way.

When you make changes, there are fresh possibilities which begin for you and your mind may be filled with weird and wonderful ideas for your next challenge. Until you reach this point, you might believe life is totally predictable. Instead, what you discover is another world opening up for you. This is a world full of unexpected delights and opportunities with plenty of fun and chances for achievements in conventional or unconventional ways.

Suddenly, things you treasure may have a new potential for you and with plenty of **encouragement**, this will be the fuel to drive you. Whatever you are passionate about is of interest to others. If you go on a charity trek in a far-off place, you might be invited to give talks about what it was like to challenge yourself in this way. Other people want to hear about what makes you 'tick', what you are enthusiastic about, who you are in your professional role or what you get up to, outside of work.

There are always some people who find it impossible to congratulate others on their achievement so you may have to **endure** comments and criticism from those who don't understand, or who are envious of you. Don't take this too personally. Be wary of these people and regard their comments as *their* problem connected with the way they see the world. Some people may be jealous of your success or maybe they don't understand what you have achieved and are too wrapped up in their own lives to be curious to find out about you. Let them go, keep connecting with your centre and be clear about what you want and where you are going.

If you start to understand what you've done and how it benefits you then move away from the complainers and avoid getting drawn into their issues. Be clear about who has the problem and separate yourself from finding their solution. Instead, connect more with those who boost your morale and fuel your excitement. They can give you the unconditional support you need, and see you and your ideas in a positive light and encourage and motivate you to take them forward. You may be surprised how simple it is to do something different once you've made up your mind and stepped over the narrow dividing line between the situation you find yourself in and the one you want.

Your 'comfort zone' may not be ideal, although it's often reassuring because you know the rules, even if you don't like them. At least it's familiar territory, and easier to cope with than to step into an unknown situation. However, crossing into your discomfort zone has the effect of increasing your comfort zone. After a short time to get used to the new you, there will be a change of attitude about what you do. What seemed difficult or even impossible will, a little while later, be automatic and usual for you.

You may be so encouraged by this that you want to do more and more and the **entrepreneur** inside of you discovers he or she is alive and well, and may want to show its face. If you have brilliant ideas which might revolutionise the way you, your colleagues or the whole world might function, you might be excited at exploring the new possibilities. If you've always had a yearning to do something innovative or unusual, you will realise that once you learn to make changes in other areas of your life you know how to take your ideas forward. Perhaps you've thought of something which could revolutionise the lives of the medical profession, for example, or for patients with certain conditions.

Don't keep these ideas to yourself. Decide what you want to explore and take a look at www.medicalfutures.co.uk. They encourage and reward innovation in doctors and support them to take these into reality. When, eventually, you take those steps, you may wonder why it took you so long. And if your ideas don't actually change the world (yet), the experience and the personal growth you experience from your exploration of them is likely to change your life. As a result, you will continue to learn and adapt the way you are in the world. Some things will work and others won't. Instead of thinking of failure regard each as a learning experience.

But the most important thing of all is to feel the **excitement** which comes from the anticipation, the planning and then the starting out on a new journey. It comes from the not knowing quite what might actually happen and from the sense that you have, at least, given it a try. All in all that might be worth the uncertainty and the fear, because of all the myriad of passions which help to fuel you onwards and upwards to the great unknown. And that might be very much more exciting than the well and truly known.

F is for

Think back to the time, many years ago when you decided you wanted to be a doctor. What was it that had the greatest influence on the decision you made back then? Perhaps you came from a medical family and it was always expected of you, or maybe you were a very good science student and your teachers encouraged you to study medicine. Maybe you were the one people used to turn to for help and advice and it seemed a natural progression for you to follow your innate desire to help people and become a doctor.

And now, how is your life compared with how you thought it would be? How is it compared with the dreams you had back then? If working in the profession has somewhat overwhelmed all the other areas of your life you may be feeling fed up from neglecting important parts of your life because work and work-related activities dominate your days.

So, if you've become aware of all of this and really want to improve things, you can start the process of change by beginning to think about your **favourite** scenario in your ideal way of life. Consider carefully what your dream might be and see it, like a video running in your mind's eye. Then imagine stepping into the scene so that you are no longer watching as an outsider, you are there experiencing it, looking around, hearing the birds sing and noticing how wonderful it is to be happy and relaxed and full of energy again. Become aware of what it's like for you being where you'd really like to be.

What's different about this scenario compared to your current life? Supposing you decide this is the place you really want to be, ask yourself what's stopping you from getting there. All sorts of things may inhibit you, such as apprehension about the unknown, or worry about what people might say about you. Even though you know what you want, the thought of actually being there and living like that may seem scary. It could be **fear** of failure, fear of making the wrong choice, or fear of not being perfect. But you don't have to be perfect,[1] though many doctors behave as though it's possible to be.

Everyone makes mistakes and it's alright to do so. An important way to learn is from your errors, so reassure yourself. It's good enough to try something even if you fail at first. Gain knowledge from your experience and try again, in a slightly different way to achieve your goals. You might even consider whether your goal is what you really want. It's not until you take some steps towards it that you may discover you have started on the wrong route. And if you've done so you can go back a few steps and take a different path. That is acceptable too, because, inevitably, as you go through life your needs change. Things which were so important to you as a teenager may not seem important at all when you reach your 30s, 40s, 50s or 60s. As you go through life your perspective changes and as your basic needs, such as having somewhere to live and finding a partner, are satisfied you may then move on to satisfy higher needs such as mentoring younger colleagues or even changing the world. Remember, what you do now doesn't have to be **forever**. It just has to be something you feel passionately about now. It must be something that you, not someone else, want to achieve.

Nevertheless, if you make any changes to hugely improve your quality of life this is a way which helps you become aware of new possibilities from which will develop your vision of the life you truly want to be living. When the time comes to change again don't berate yourself for past decisions, which were right for you then, in the light of your available knowledge and experience. Accept that what you did then was right for you, at the time and in relation to your circumstances.

However, if you still carry anger or resentment in relation to something which happened years ago, then ask yourself what you need to do to enable yourself to let it go and move on. Be prepared to **forgive** yourself and others for what you consider now was a wrong decision. Bear in mind that whatever people do, it is usually done with good intentions from their perspective, influenced by their circumstances and beliefs of the era.

Sometimes **friends** offer you support and encouragement and at other times all they do is criticise. Since they are important people in your life don't dismiss what they say. Nevertheless, listen fully, notice their concerns and also that many of these concerns are not really much about you. They are actually more about themselves and how they believe your plan will impact on them. Acknowledge their concerns and then remind yourself of the reasons for wanting to change your life and why you want to make your own decisions about this.

However, if what you want is **fulfilment** in life and you want your life to be more balanced so you can have time for a social life away from work colleagues, to be with your partner, your family, friends and community, with time to do things by yourself too, then you have to decide how you will make the changes to accomplish these things.

If you hope for a different **future** then you know, if you do nothing, that in a few years' time your situation may be as it is now, or even busier, more stressful, with more work and less time for outside activities. Remember, nothing much changes in your life if all you do is think, 'I don't want so and so any more'.

An important part of making changes is identifying what you want, rather than concentrating on what you don't want. It's about turning your visions into achievable goals, and taking the actions to move forward bit by bit in the direction you want to go. Since the more you think about what you would like, the more likely it is to happen then spending time thinking, dreaming and planning your strategies for change are all valuable things to be doing – not just thinking about, but also experiencing, in your imagination, your ideal scenario. So as well as what your ideal life looks like, think too of what it smells and sounds like and also become aware of your mood and emotions.

In order to shift from where you are to where you want to be, you have several options. Some may be obvious, some not so. You could start by writing down all the possible ways in which you might move towards the life you really want and then notice which option resonates most with you. Explore this first. Don't dismiss any of the alternatives out of hand, but challenge yourself instead. Ask yourself 'why?' to each objection you make. If you really want the realisation of your dreams then you have to take that leap of faith and start with a small step. Until you do something differently, nothing changes. So, take a deep breath and either jump or step gently from your comfort zone to your discomfort zone. When you do, you may be surprised to find that not only does what seemed so scary and difficult seem much easier, but also that your comfort zone increases enormously.

Reference

1 Kersley S (2003) Can you let go of being perfect? *BMJ Career Focus.* **327**: S76.

G is for

Goal	**Grounding**
Good enough	**Growth**
Gratitude	**Guilt**
Greatness	

Some people use too much energy complaining about how overworked they are, how tired they are, or how they would do things if they were managing the health service; all that energy expended and not much left either to get on and do what has to be done or to explore and discover new ways to approach the challenges. If you are frustrated by the way your life never seems to change, then you have to take some action. You need to develop a strategy and timetable for the way you want to make those changes.

But, the very first thing to do is to be clear about what you *do want* rather than focusing entirely on what you *don't want.* When you do this your centre of attention is on your dreams and aspirations rather than on your stresses and strains. When you are able to clearly identify a positive and precise **goal** you will be better able to define the steps you must take to move yourself towards it.

Too many people don't change because all they do is talk about what's wrong with the system and what someone else has to do to make it better. You may be waiting a long time for that to happen. When you've decided on a desired outcome, ask yourself if it is reasonable or are you being idealistic about your desired end result. Check in with yourself and make sure your aim is what *you* really want, rather than what someone else has told you is what is best for you now. Make sure it is what *you* would reasonably be able to accomplish if you have enough support and encouragement.

If you are certain about these things, you can progress to making plans and deciding how to progress with your project. If you tend to want everything to be perfect and usually procrastinate because you think it wouldn't be as good as it could be, just yet, then consider that there always is a balance between perfection and accomplishing something **good enough**, i.e. going for the silver rather than the gold standard. Surely it is better to do this even if it is not completely faultless, than not do anything at all.

Make your goal manageable so that it will be one you can expect to reach in a reasonable time. In this way you will experience success rather than failure. This might mean deciding to go for an interim goal at first. Then you will move easily towards your bigger objective, step by step, and will gradually move nearer and nearer towards it. You may not be able to go home an hour earlier immediately but as you work faster and more resourcefully you may make a difference each day of five minutes, so that after a couple of weeks you would achieve your desired outcome.

Doing this will have a wider effect too. You will work more efficiently, have more time to relax at home, begin to enjoy your social life much more and experience fun and enjoyment again engaging with hobbies you almost forgot about. Succeeding is empowering and the **gratitude** you feel towards those who helped and encouraged you along the way enables you to set another goal to move yourself forward even more. Not only that, but also when you appreciate how much someone has helped you with their support, you are more likely to enjoy giving support to others and helping them make their life transformations too.

If sometimes you are beset by feelings of failure, of not being able to do what you want, you are not alone. However, it is important to be realistic and recognise your potential. Don't allow your internal critic to rule your life. Yes, that critical voice, whether inside yourself or from others, is important because it enables you to realise what might go wrong and may bring you back to earth with questions and doubts about your plans.

When you think about what might happen you could decide on plan B as a back up to use if the worst scenario actually took place. However it's important not to let the critical voice stop you from carrying out your plans. Yes, listen to what it says and then counterbalance those comments with your voice of reason because that will let you know how to overcome any obstacles which might occur. If you expand rather than diminish your beliefs about what you can achieve, you have **greatness** beyond anything you can envisage.

> *Our deepest fear is not that we are inadequate. Our deepest fear is that we are powerful beyond measure. It is our Light, not our Darkness, that most frightens us. We ask ourselves, who am I to be brilliant, gorgeous, talented, and fabulous? Actually, who are you NOT to be? You are a child of God. Your playing small does not serve the world.*[1]

Do you recall the ritual humiliation of the ward round when you were a medical student or junior doctor? Do you remember times when you've been told off in front of a patient for forgetting to arrange a special blood test or for not having the appropriate X-ray available? How often have you been reprimanded for something you did wrong compared with how rarely someone in the medical work situation says 'Well done, you did a great job'? Wouldn't it be empowering to be praised more often for a job well done?

If you prefer praise rather than criticism then start to compliment others more frequently, because a great principle for initiating change is the realisation that the way you are towards others is reflected by the way they behave towards you. For instance, if you come back from a meeting and say the people there were all really unfriendly, think back and consider your own behaviour and whether you might have been more friendly towards others.

So, observe what happens when you are more generous and complimentary in your remarks and how this is reflected back in the way people behave towards you. Begin to notice the language you use and how you make statements as if they were fact when actually it's just your idea about a situation, without any **grounding** or real evidence. You may be voicing an opinion about someone based on your brief experience. 'She's lazy', you say because she didn't join in when people were asked to help put the chairs away. You made a judgement when you might not have realised she was exhausted from a weekend on-call. You could begin to challenge assumptions you and others make. On what basis do they say that you could never achieve what you want to do? On what evidence do you state that you don't have the right skills, or do you assume you wouldn't be able to acquire them?

When you act towards others as you would like them to treat you, your personal and emotional **growth** may astonish you, more than you ever imagined might be possible. You will amaze not only those around you, but yourself too, when you achieve what you set your mind to and have the support you need. It almost doesn't matter in what area of your life you set yourself a challenge.

You find that succeeding in something you set out to do impacts on the rest of your life. You may find yourself feeling guilty about moving on, letting go or changing the way you do things. You may feel responsible for other people's anger in relation to what you do. If you want the life you could have then learn to let go of the **guilt** and start to do something for yourself, knowing that it's alright to put yourself first for a change.

Putting yourself first is about self-care and self-esteem. It's about enabling you to look after yourself. You will then be better able to fulfil your obligations to others and everyone benefits not only you.

Reference

1 Williamson M (1992) *A Return To Love*. Harper Collins, London.

H is for

Habitual	**Heart**
Handle	**Help**
Happiness	**Holistic**
Head	**Hope**
Health	

When you started your job as a fresh-faced keen doctor, ready and eager to learn the routines of the practice or ways to complete ward rounds efficiently, you may have been shown the ropes by your partners or by someone else in the team. They will have told you what has to be done and explained how to do it. And from that day on until today you followed their guidance impeccably, just doing it all, rarely questioning, getting through the routine tasks of the day.

Begin to notice how you have a way of dealing with situations in a **habitual** way, the way you were taught years ago. Those ways may not be the most efficient nowadays and you may not even realise that there are other possibilities which could open up when you begin to **handle** a situation differently. Unless you take some time to observe yourself, what you do and how you feel when doing those things, for a few days, you will remain stuck in those routines.

When you take time to notice how you spend your day, how you approach what you do and the way you have for doing it, then there may be obvious changes for the better which you could make. Maybe you don't realise how your mood affects the way you cope. You might become aware of how much longer you take to do those things you don't like doing. If you resent some things and enjoy others, notice how your efficiency changes in relation to those emotions.

When you appreciate times when you are happy, then you become aware of what has to change in your life so that you can experience **happiness** more often. To get through your day more effectively, consider ways to lighten the tasks which weigh you down. Could you delegate those? Do your colleagues do them more quickly?

How do they do that? It's usually very helpful to ask and observe those who do things differently because you may discover ways to change your own ways too. Notice how you feel when things are going well, when you are enjoying your day and working effectively without stress. Do you have a sense of joy, of bliss, of delight or of contentment or is there just the absence of unhappiness?

Did you know that it's possible to condition yourself to a positive mind-set whenever you want to? Just like Pavlov with his dog, you can train yourself to experience a desired emotion in response to an anchoring stimulus, such as pressing your forefinger and thumb together. If you do this each time you feel, for example, great happiness (or even just recall an intense feeling of happiness), or whatever emotion you wish to have, then you will be able to experience the emotion whenever you want to, in response to this small physical movement. This technique is a useful one for coping with day-to-day tasks, and even for dealing with difficult patients or colleague.

Decide on the emotion you want to be able to access in a certain situation, recall a time when you experienced it very intensely and anchor it, so that you have it available as and when you want it.

If you tend to be a left brain sort of person who deals with situations very logically and tends to live in your **head**, then it may change your perception of the world if you can connect much more with your emotional side. This is about connecting more with your right brain creative side, and recognising too how the world is experienced not only in your head but also in your body.

Becoming more aware of any tense areas, and consciously taking a deep breath into them in order to relax any tense muscles, is useful as a way of understanding and learning how to deal with a stressful situation more effectively. As a result of doing this you can develop ways to make the changes you want in your routine, in your day and in your life.

If work dominates your existence, takes up most of your time, and a great deal of your emotional and physical energy, you may not be looking after your physical and emotional **health** as well as you could. If you always make excuses in relation to being too busy and say you don't have the time or the energy to take some regular exercise, or can't be bothered to eat more healthy food, to stop smoking or drink less alcohol, then just stop right there.

If you want to transform your life, the basics are important. Don't neglect them. Are you living a well-balanced, fulfilled and happy life?[1] You could make the decision, as from today, to look after your body, mind and spirit much more. Since these are interconnected, something such as exercise will have an effect on them all. When you do this, you will notice a positive impact on the way you cope with your life and your **heart** will sing again!

Are you someone who wants to do everything yourself, i.e. a bit of a control freak? Someone who can't stand asking for **help,** because only you know how to do it properly? Isn't it time now to review this mind-set and recognise that it's useful to talk to others and do more things together? Think of it as a way to free up some time in order to do the 'looking after yourself' things you want to do, rather than any sign of weakness.

Because, when you take a **holistic** view of your life, you may begin to realise you are more than a doctor. The doctor label sticks very hard, but really, you *are* more than your work. You are more than all the parts of yourself and your life. They are interconnected and valuable. Stop neglecting the parts you've been forgetting. It's important to have a life too. It's essential to have time away from not only your place of work but also the briefcase full of patient files taken home each night.

Although being a doctor may be regarded by some as more than a job, does it have to be an overwhelming lifestyle too? Remember, there is more to life than your work; you are a person too. You are entitled, like any other human being to have time for yourself, for a partner, for friends, family and community. Don't let those needs be swallowed up by the needs of your profession. Perhaps you realise that some of your important desires, such as status, success and self-esteem are met through your work.

Maybe it would be worth reflecting on how important these are to you and if they are what you want. How else could you satisfy them in ways apart from your role as a doctor? Which parts of your life are you neglecting by putting so much of your time and energy into your working life?

Think about how your life can be fulfilled in ways apart from through your work. Make a resolution to find, without any further delay, regular time for family, friends, your partner and your community and, most importantly, yourself.

Which part of your life needs more attention? If you look after all aspects of your life on a regular basis then your experience of happiness may increase.[2] You will be able to look forward to the future with **hope**, secure in the knowledge that it will be the one you want.

References

1 Kersley S (2001) Striking the balance. *BMJ Career Focus.* **323:** S2.

2 Kersley S (2003) Wellbeing: reality or dream? *BMJ Career Focus.* **326:** S109.

I is for

Identity	**Integrate**
Imagination	**Integrity**
Impatience	**Internal dialogue**
Inkling	**Intuition**

Have you ever been at a conference or social event and someone asks, 'Where are you from?'. What does the question mean for you? Do you say where you live now, where you grew up, where you lived as a child, where you were born, where your parents were born or where your grandparents were born? Another question which is related but different is 'Where are you coming from?'. You might be asked this in a situation where there may be some disagreement or when it is hoped to proceed with a project in some harmony. The question is to find out something about your beliefs and values, about what's important to you, what life has taught you about the nature of men, of women, of relationships, of this, of that . . .? So, who exactly are *you*?

What is *your* true **identity?** You are made up of so many diverse parts and each of these and more can have some bearing on and affect your thoughts and behaviour today. Some of the pressures on you may be very strong and yet you may not even be aware of how powerful they are in impinging on the way you are in the world. As you begin to think more deeply about these things you may begin to realise and understand how some of them may have had a very strong influence on you and how until now you may have been living a life to fulfil someone else's expectations for you. As you find out more about yourself, what excites and drives you, you start to define more clearly what *you* truly want for the rest of your life, even if it's something different from the wishes of those near and dear to you.

Imagination is an important tool which is a way to develop yourself and decide how you want to change. It enables you to find out more about what you need to look after yourself more and to expand your ideas to take you forward. Without imagination it may be difficult to be clear about what your transformed life might be, especially if you tend to think more in negative terms of what you don't want, which is all very well up to a point, but it isn't easy to know where to go from there. When all you think about is what you want to move away from, you may find it difficult to make changes because you need to have something to aim for. However, when you start to day-dream and think very carefully about what you desire, then things start to shift. When you take time to picture your new life in more and more detail, noticing colours, whether what you see is near or far, and playing around with bringing it more into focus, nearer or brighter, to find the best representation you can, then the more likely it is to happen.

You may find you tune in more to the sounds and smells of what you want, or find that what really connects with you are the feelings you have when you know you will soon reach your dream in your true existence. By letting go of your **impatience** and doing this exercise in a relaxed and quiet way and then writing and reflecting on what you discover is likely to be extremely useful. Imagination can take you from a place of not knowing to a place of clarity.

As you think about your possible ways forward you may suddenly be aware of something inside you, an **inkling**, an internal reaction of knowing, when you understand exactly what you must do to solve the challenge or problem you've been deliberating about for ages. This happens when you relax and let ideas flow into your head without editing and without comment. Just notice what happens. This process can help you **integrate**, i.e. join together your present reality with your desired future with honesty and **integrity**. It helps you move from 'no more of this' to 'this is what I want'. You will remain true to yourself, your beliefs, your values and your morals. It's about being who you are and making changes which fit for you, in a way and at a time when it's right for you. When you do, you will notice a difference in the way you view life and what impacts on you. Some things which previously you might have reacted to with anger or frustration may seem less important, because you begin to realise and put into practice the idea that you can choose your reaction to something. Instead of anger you could choose action; instead of frustration you could choose acceptance. Until you are able to live in harmony and congruence with your truth then you may remain dissatisfied and frustrated with your life. This is about getting back to the very basics of your life, your true foundation.

Start with yourself. Review the code and rules which dominate your actions and ask yourself if these are the ones you want or if it is time to move on. Do you need to upgrade some and get rid of others? Is this the moment to reaffirm and renew your commitment to moving from where you come from to where you are going? Is it time to renew your undertaking to be who you truly want to be? Consider whether it's time to reassess what is really essential in your life and what fits with your authenticity.

Real integrity is doing the right thing, knowing that nobody's going to know whether you did it or not.

Oprah Winfrey

If you are on the brink of making a huge change and wonder whether or not to take a leap into something new you may be wondering how you decide what action to take or what to actually do differently. This time of confusion is a time to tune in to your **internal dialogue**, the secret conversations with yourself that criticise or tell you what you should or shouldn't do. As you consider the various ways you might proceed, notice how you feel as you consider each one. Is there one which seems to call out to you, or do you get a strong feeling about another, or is there a vivid picture of how things might be? Notice these things and notice too what you tell yourself and then ask 'who said so?' or 'why? – or even 'why not?'.

Observe how often you make assumptions about people's thoughts or situations. You may talk as if you can mind-read but check out your theories, you may be wrong. Be aware of whether your opinions are predominately negative. Have a go at changing them to be more positive and notice what happens. Allow your heart to guide you as much as your head. Trust your **intuition**, your sixth sense, your gut feeling about something. Notice what happens to you when you consider your different options. Be aware of your reaction as you think about each one. Make the choice based on which one gives you a buzz, or an insight into what is best and then take action!

J is for

Jealousy	**Judgemental**
Journey	**Juggle**
Judgement	**Juxtaposition**

When you look around at your colleagues do you ever feel a twinge of **jealousy** about those who seem to have their life 'sorted'? Do they always finish on time, always look smart and efficient and seem to cope with the workload much better than you do? What is their secret? Do they really deal with it all better than you, or are you making superficial judgements based on scant evidence. You never really know what life is like for the other person, or how they experience the same situation, unless you talk to each other about it. You may be surprised by what they say to you.

First of all they may tell you how good at coping with the workload you appear to be too. You may not even realise how you appear to others and how they make assumptions about you too. Ask your apparently more proficient than you colleague to explain and demonstrate what they actually do. Get them to tell it to you step by tiny step so that you can begin to understand them better. Do this rather than assuming that you already know. It's the best way to learn. Sometimes you spend so long trying to understand something from books you forget there are practical skills you need too. Experts don't always do something as it was taught to them. They find ways to adapt the principles so they carry out the procedure in a way which works for them.

Notice how simple things can be done in lots of different ways. For example, there are many different ways to make a cup of tea. You may be surprised to find out alternative ways to do what you've been doing as a routine for a long time. And changing the way you do something is the starting point for changing much, much more.

Life is often compared to a **journey**. First you think about where you might like to go; you consider the features and the pros and cons of the various destinations. You decide if you want to go a long way or just a short distance. But before you move on to booking the transport and somewhere to stay, you have to come to a definite decision. You have to know where you are going. You have to know your destination in order to plan how to get there and with whom you want to make the journey, or whether you prefer to travel alone. You must remind yourself too the purpose of your journey and why you want to be somewhere else, instead of where you are now. Then you will find the maps so that you can book the right transport and follow the correct route to get there.

However, you may discover new opportunities on the way and decide to change your plans and go down a different road, or you may remain very focused on your original direction. Sometimes, being willing to explore highways and byways is very useful because you discover new possibilities. Are you staying on the path you started on? Do you know there are other ways to explore? That's up to you to decide as you travel along it. If you believe a diversion might be interesting find out where it goes; it may lead you to your desired destination. If not you can go back. You are not a hamster on a wheel; you can get off and rest and reassess the situation whenever you want.

How can you use your **judgement**, to decide if your path is the right one for you, or if you need to follow a different route? You could notice and monitor how you are from day to day and even from hour to hour. Notice when you feel elated and happy and how often you have a sense of fulfilment. Notice too what you are doing when you are tense or stressed and how your body changes compared with when you are happy and fulfilled. What happens to your mood when you change your body and relax areas of tension? If you find yourself saying to yourself 'I hate doing that' then you will. If instead you change your thoughts to something like 'I'm relaxed and enjoying whatever I do today' then you will change the way you experience your day.

If you are uncertain about whether to continue as you are or to change your path, then start by making a list of the pros and cons of each direction you are considering. Try to view each alternative without being too **judgemental**. Sometimes the least likely path turns out to be the way you really want to go. As you do this you may find that the right way for you becomes obvious. If it doesn't you could toss a coin to give you the answer. Notice your reaction and then ignore what the coin tells you and choose to do what excites and interests you instead.

You may want to delay until you know this way or that way is definitely the right direction. You may assume it's possible to know these things. Generally, it's not. You have to take the chance, go where you think is the right way and then review and assess. And if it's not right, go for the next option. It's noticing what goes well and what doesn't, and deciding whether or not to stick with it for longer or to let it go and move on. It's about life, the universe and learning by trial and error. It's also about realising that some-times it's worth persisting and not giving up too soon, if you really want to achieve something which is important to you. Think of a little child learning to walk and not giving up the first time they fall over. When hassle from others annoys you take a deep breath and keep centred. Don't let their behaviour push you over.

When your own need for change becomes overwhelming and pulls you in the opposite direction, you have to keep calm and **juggle** the demands made on your time and energy, while recognising that this is a temporary phase, part of your experience of change. Just like the circus performer, if you have too many plates in the air some will inevitably fall. So decide what you can stop spinning. Which **juxtaposition** of activities is no longer viable for you?

Which of your plates can you let go?

K is for

Kaleidoscope	**Kinaesthetic**
Keenness	**Kindle**
Keeping fit	**Kith and kin**
Kick-start	**Knowledge**

You could compare life to a **kaleidoscope** because it, too, has infinite possibilities and endless variations, of how it can be. When you give it just a little shake, the pattern changes completely. These changing patterns, some beautiful, others less so, are as the pieces of your life might be rearranged too. It depends on whether you can take a chance to shake it, just a little, and notice what happens. The new pattern may be big or small, colourful or plain. When the pattern becomes clearer, you can decide if this is the one you want in your life now or if you want to change it more. Whatever it is, you will know when it's the right pattern because you will have a sense of **keenness** about you and what you want in your life.

When you look back to the time you decided to study medicine, did you realise how much of your personal time might be eroded, swallowed up by medical work? This is not only by the time it takes to see and treat your patients but also by the time taken for studying, the administration, the government directives, the meetings and the research. The amount of work may seem almost endless and yet you have to get through it somehow or other with varying degrees of urgency. You may find you are so busy you forget, or don't attend to the importance of **keeping fit**. This is vital for the wellbeing of your body, mind and spirit. When you look after yourself properly you are likely to be so much better at caring for others. Instead of being tired and irritable you will have renewed 'get-up-and-go' to cope with your work, and have the energy to consider how to change things too.

Recognising your own needs as a person is vital. Nevertheless, however healthy your lifestyle, remember and recognise that, in spite of being a doctor, you too can become ill sometimes. If you feel under the weather or notice lumps and bumps which you know shouldn't be there seek appropriate advice and treatment. Don't self-medicate. Don't ask your colleague for a quick piece of advice in a busy corridor. Look after yourself in the way which you would advise another doctor or any other patient. When you are poorly enough to take time away from work, take the time to fully recover. Don't go back until you are well again. To embark on a new way of life you need to be at your most fit.

If you want to **kick-start** your fitness then take a look at yourself from another perspective. Start with the basics for good health. It's easy to be complacent about the food you eat and the amount of physical exercise you take. Try stepping out of yourself and think about how you and your lifestyle might appear to an impartial observer. What advice or suggestions would they make to you? With these insights perhaps you could set yourself a routine to gradually improve your health and wellbeing.

How do you think about your future, living your ideal life? People vary in the way they do this. If you mainly think about it in pictures, you are, in the main, a visual person. If you tend to think more about sounds or what is said, your thinking style is auditory. If you are someone who is, for the most part, aware of feelings then your style is **kinaesthetic**. You tap into the emotions you will have when you reach your goal. However, most people have a bit of each of these styles, although often there is one which is predominant.

When you make changes in your life other unexpected opportunities open up for you and you begin to **kindle** new interests. These might be in areas about which you were previously unaware. You may discover you have a skill which can be used in different ways. So, give yourself permission to explore those things which inspire you and enjoy the new paths which open up for you as a result.

Stop saying 'One day, when I've got the time, I'd love to . . .', and instead plan to do whatever it is, now, or in the very near future. When you've dismissed any goals which truly are unrealistic or unachievable by you (not setting your ambitions too low) then almost anything else you want to do is possible, once you set your mind to it. By deciding on a clear goal and the steps you must take to reach it, you have to take the first step and then you are on the way. Tell yourself it's alright to do something differently. In the end, it's not the doing that's difficult, it's the thoughts in your head, about it, which may stop you.

You may be reluctant to put your plans into practice because of worries about your perception of the effects of the changes on your nearest and dearest. Your family, friends and colleagues, your **kith and kin**, who are all used to you behaving in a certain way, may be shocked or surprised when you do or say something different, and they may do their best to discourage you from continuing. They may not understand why you want to change your life. They may believe their lives might change for the worse as a result of your proposed action, and think you are making a big mistake. Maybe they're right and maybe they're wrong. How can you know until you do it? Bear in mind that they have their own agenda which may not be congruent with yours. Because they love and care about you, they don't want you to be hurt or upset if your plans fail.

However, sometimes the resistance you think you will encounter is not borne out by experience. It may be in your head. You may imagine you can read their minds and think you know how others will react to you, but that's not true. So, what can you do to have as much co-operation as possible?

- Be really clear about what you want.
- Set specific goals.
- Don't make assumptions about other people.
- Be positive about the benefits your change will bring not only to you but to them too. Then they could be your best advocates and applaud and support you in your new endeavour.
- Acquire the skills and knowledge you need.

Life-long learning is essential, whether for continuing professional development or learning more about the things you love. When you stop learning you stop living.

Most of all be ready to go out into the world with a sense of curiosity and a thirst for new **knowledge**. By recognising you don't know something by saying 'I don't know' is the first step to learning and means you are ready to do so. You will be ready to experience new patterns in your life.

L is for

Language	**Limbic**
Learn	**Listen**
Let go	**Loss**
Lightness	**Love**

When you go about your daily tasks talking to patients, colleagues, friends and family you are probably hardly aware of the strength of, not only the choice of words you use, but also how you frame what you say. Do you know that one of the greatest tools for changing your life at your disposal, is your use of **language**?

When you talk to someone about what you want to do and express your ideas in certain ways, then your world begins to change. The more you become aware of the power of language, the more you realise how you may tend to make huge assumptions about others or about a situation. When you say something as though it is a fact, it may be your opinion rather than provable. Notice what you and others say about a situation or a person and then imagine stepping back and asking, 'How do I know that to be true?'. Whether or not something is true, it may be believed as 'the way things are' when actually it is someone's opinion. Whether what you say is true or not, stating it can make it seem to be correct. Yet when you search for evidence there may be none, except for several people saying something. Passing on other people's comments begins to form an assumption of truth.

As an example of how language alters action, notice what happens in a scenario when someone asks you do them a favour. Depending on whether you say 'I'll do it' or 'No, I don't want to do it', you will have created something different. Your language will have changed your behaviour.

If you realise you've been guilty of spreading information about someone without any clear information to back it up, don't worry. Just consider what you might do differently another time. If bearing a grudge against someone bothers you, even though it might be related to an incident which happened ages ago then think about it and ask yourself, 'What did I **learn** from that?'.

Since turning the clock back is not possible, you could instead decide to change your mind-set.

- Remove blame from what you or they did or said.
- Let the picture in your mind of what happened fade from colour to black and white, from large to small, from loud to silent.

Sometimes you have to release resentment, **let go** of anger and be willing to move on. When you decide to do this then new possibilities become more likely, if you are ready and open to them. Don't let resentments from the past prevent you from being in the right frame of mind now.

Perhaps you tend to take past events far too seriously and hold resentment for longer than you need to. It may help to develop another way of looking at past events. Try thinking about some events which in the past upset you, with some **lightness**. Find a way to tell the story about what happened; recall with humour. Have a laugh about it! Try retelling the events in a positive way or fictionalise them as a story. You could have a go at turning it into a fairy story or a detective yarn or romantic tale. You won't deny what happened, however it helps you to move on and place the event into your past personal biography rather than in the present, and you will be better able to look forward with new excitement to life as it unfolds before you.

As you tell your story to someone who understands where you are coming from, and demonstrates empathy, you are probably experiencing **limbic** resonance, the primitive, unconscious connection made between two people 'in tune' with each other. This happens to their physiology too, as heart rates become similar. Whatever it is, it happens and when it does magic happens.

Learning to really **listen** is so important in communication. Deep listening is about not only what is said but what isn't too. It's about allowing a space to let the person who is speaking process the information thoroughly and so come to a new understanding of their situation. Don't jump in too quickly with what you think the person wants. Check with them. Allow some silences. These give space for processing and contemplation.

When someone tells you all that is wrong with their life, you don't have to solve everything for them. If you feel overwhelmed by a 'heart-sink' patient who goes on and on with endless problems, you don't have to sort them all out in the short time they have for their appointment. Ask what they want from you today. Listen to the answer. It may be something quite straight-forward such as 'Please sign this form'. You can breathe a sigh of relief. You don't have to sort out everything for them.

When people talk, they don't always want solutions. Sometimes what they want is someone who listens, really listens, to them. Being heard may be a luxury. Too often you start to speak and the listener jumps in with the reply they think you expect. As a doctor, do you notice how often you hear a few symptoms and your mind has already decided to prescribe those tablets or arrange that blood test. And because you have a waiting room full of patients, this may be the strategy which works for you to enable you to get through the day.

Notice what happens when you let go of solutions and listen and acknowledge. This enables the other person to find their own answer and express what they want. Change is not always painless or straightforward. It may involve you in sleepless nights and much soul-searching. Nearly every change, however much achieving it will improve your life, involves some grieving too. Change is often about **loss** of some sort. It might be loss of a job or a home, or loss of a long-held identity. It seems as though this is part of moving on to something different.

Change is also about bringing an increasing **love** of others and most of all a love of yourself more into your life. Have you ever looked into your own eyes in the mirror and told yourself 'I love you'. Try it some time and observe how that feels. When you come from a place of love, everything fits. The secret of loving other people is to first love yourself.

M is for

Magical	**Mind map**
Magician	**Mood**
Mentor	**Movement**
Metaphor	

Do you remember the time when you believed in the magic that happened in stories and wondered if fairies and elves lived at the bottom of the garden? Perhaps you've become rather cynical about things happening with little reason, and always want someone to tell you why or how something comes to pass. Explanation works well in the world of science and medicine, most of the time, except when things occur for which there doesn't seem to be any logic. Perhaps a patient recovered when you thought there was little hope, and for a fleeting moment you wondered if there was some magic in the air. It's quite exhilarating to let go of needing to know 'why' and just for a while, to accept the way things turn out. Certainly, when you decide to change your life and take the first tentative steps towards something different, then something **magical** may happen. It's as if the world itself changes too. People and places seem unlike the way they were before, and it becomes easier to believe that what you hope for might actually be possible.

When you were a child you may have met a special person at a party, a **magician**. You were baffled by rabbits coming out of hats and by bunches of flowers appearing from nowhere. Sometimes, when you decide to make changes you will meet another sort of magician. They may have come into your life unexpectedly and be there at the right time for you – someone who seems to understand what's driving you, someone you can bounce your ideas onto, someone who gives you a helping hand, a phone number or two or something magic, such as asking you a challenging question or two which hits the spot absolutely and as a result you have a flash of inspiration or fantastic insight.

During a time of life change it's motivating and useful to have a coach or **mentor** to be the magician in your life. What you achieve by working with your personal magician may be quite remarkable and unexpected. It can make a world of difference to have someone to support you during your period of transition. Working with a mentor or a coach is a good way to reduce overwhelm and the procrastination you may encounter when you decide to make changes in your life.

Perhaps, if you are a mentor yourself, you may be part of one of many mentoring schemes.[1] If so, make sure you work with your own mentor too. It's useful to experience, for yourself, the benefit mentoring brings. Everyone gains as a result, not only your mentees but also, most of all, yourself. You'll find out at first hand how beneficial it is to have someone to offload onto about things which are challenging in your life.

When new concepts are difficult to understand then a powerful way to move an idea forward is by using **metaphor** to compare something with similar attributes to the subject you are considering. For example, the changing seasons of the year are useful as a metaphor in relation to how you feel about aspects of your life and may help you understand how the process for change happens internally.[2] If you are considering leaving something, you may feel like Autumn moving towards Winter. Then you may experience a time when outwardly things are dormant and you lack energy and drive. However, inwardly things are happening. When your Spring arrives you have more energy, new hope. It is a period for growth and anticipation. Quite suddenly, it seems, you are filled with ideas and energy. You are ready to take the first steps for change. Finally, you move into Summer and your life is in full bloom again.

A very useful tool, for initiating and planning change, is the **mind map**. It is a superb way to discover what to do in a challenging situation. Devised by Tony Buzan,[3] mind maps are an effective technique to use even at a most simple level. With the subject of your challenge or deliberation written in the centre of your paper, draw radiating lines with the topics which arise from them. You can use different colours and sketches in addition to words to represent each heading.

The mind map is a snapshot of your thoughts and gets you away from the usual listing which leads to prioritising in a linear way. You have a representation of your reflection on the subject on one piece of paper. The method gets you to think 'outside of the box' and gives you the opportunity to notice links between different parts of your map. This is more difficult to do when you make lists, because these tend to make you believe the things at the top are more important than those further down.

When you've used a tool such as a mind map, it's interesting to notice how your **mood** changes as you explore your various options. Get out of your head again and identify where you feel something in your body as you consider your life. When you draw your mind map notice which bits seem to fire you up and which areas seem to be connected with no energy. Whatever your mind-set or emotion, you can change things instantly by changing your body. When you take a more open or flexible stance become aware of how different your mood becomes. This may be to do with your posture or taking a bit more exercise. Some people find that going for a swim or dancing to lively music helps to change the way they feel in themselves and also about something they are considering.

Movement is very important, too, because it changes your energy levels and your mood. If you are fed up, notice how much better you feel after some exercise. The way you walk may reflect your internal feelings. Notice any areas of tension or stiffness when you walk, take a deep breath and relax those areas.

Have a look at how others walk. Everyone has their own style. It can be a bit of fun when you walk behind someone and, without them noticing, try to walk like they do. You may find an insight into how differently they view the world from you. Play around with observing how others move, try copying them for a while and notice how walking differently changes the way you feel. There is a relationship between these three things: if your mood changes so then does your language and body too. A change in one affects the other two. When you realise this you can change what seems easiest to you and watch what happens to the other two.

References

1 Bowen-Simpkins P, Mellows H and Dhillon C (2004) Royal College of Obstetricians and Gynaecologists Mentoring Scheme. BMJ Career Focus. **328**: 56–60.

2 McClelland C (1998) *Seasons of Change: Using nature's wisdom to grow through life's inevitable ups and downs.* Conari Press, Berkeley, CA.

3 Buzan T (2003) *How to Mind Map: Make the most of your mind and learn how to create, organise and plan.* Harper Collins, London.

N for

Needs	**New**
Negative	**New Life**
Networking	**No**

If your life until now has been one job after another with very little time to draw breath in between, with pressure to apply for the next post to look good on your CV, then you may not have taken a moment to step back and see yourself, your life and how on earth you got onto the treadmill from which you think you are about to fall or be pushed. Have you ever considered what drives you? Have you ever considered what your job brings you apart from the income? Could it be status and self-esteem? Could it be success and money? Could it be security and self-satisfaction? Is your very being validated by the work you do? Whether you like it or not, if the thought of changing the way you work, or the sort of work you do, scares you so much that you do nothing about it, then you may be tapping into how your work fulfils something very important for you.

These are your **needs** which are so compelling they absolutely have to be met one way or another. Many of yours may be met by your occupation and be a cause of your unrelenting busyness. It's worth taking some time to think about how these needs might be fulfilled in other ways, because until you discover this you may find that making changes is almost impossible.

If you live in a mainly **negative** frame of mind, and are certain without further thought that nothing can be changed, so it's futile to try, then that will be your experience. If you feel that no one else could possibly do your job, you remain stuck where you are. If you are not happy in your day-to-day life than something has to change. It may be the way you organise your working day rather than changing it completely.

Talking to others doing similar jobs can be really useful. Apart from talking to people you know already, consider attending events at which **networking** is possible. It's a great way to expand your life possibilities because the more people you talk to, the more likely you are to find out about different ways of doing things, and ways to get out of your rut.

As a result of various conversations, you might hear about and decide to explore something **new**, which you might not have considered before. It's useful to talk to someone who has followed a similar path and find out what worked and what didn't work for them. You will be better able to make your own choices as a result.

You could question some of the ways things are, if they aren't working well. The challenge for you is differentiating what truly cannot be changed and not reaching that conclusion too quickly. Then you can be more sure about what can or can't be changed, and take the action that has to be taken. There are often other ways to do things if you are willing to discover them. Then you begin to make a difference to your life. In the end it depends on you, whether you've genuinely had enough of your present situation and want to enter a **new life**, and you want to find the way to move towards it.

When you start this process of reflection and exploration, you may find your life has been taken over by the demands of your work so much that you find it really difficult to set boundaries and say **no**. If this has happened to you, then take a stand, today, and decide you won't put up with the situation any longer. Instead, recognise that now is the time to re-visit hobbies and things which made your heart sing in the past. Doing this is as important as having oxygen to breathe or enough food to eat. Discover once more the person behind your professional role.

How can you say *no* when you usually say *yes*? It's very difficult to say you can't do something if you are the sort of person who wants to be wanted and who likes to be liked. The person asking you the favour may well have asked several others before you. You might learn from their ability to say 'no'. When you say 'yes' when you really are too busy then what you do is to dismiss the importance of self-care. There is only a certain amount you can reasonably do during the working day, so be aware of this and don't overstep your mark. Also, don't dismiss your own time as unimportant. Some people consider that working part time means you have time free to do more work for them. Make the time for you and your activities as protected and important as the times for surgeries or ward rounds. Avoid the trap of giving lots of excuses, just respond to a request by saying, 'No, I can't do that, I have to do something else'. Beware of giving excuses which my be counter-balanced by the person asking you to do something. You can pad it out, if you like, by saying, 'Thank you for asking me to do this. However, I'm very sorry but I'm unable to do it at this time because I have a lot of other commitments. Thanks again for thinking of me'. If you want to change but find it difficult, ask yourself, what needs are being met by staying put. You can then decide to get these needs met in another way. Use a mind map to discover how to do this.

You may not want to hear this but, perhaps, if you work hard and long hours, it's a way to avoid being with your family, friends and community, or you may use work as an excuse not to look after yourself as well as you could, or to avoid any social life. Do you blame the system, conveniently forgetting that the system eventually changes because of individuals who make a difference?

By taking some small action you can begin to change things not only for you, but for all the other people who are affected by your change.

O is for

Obstacles	**Options**
Openness	**Original**
Opportunities	**Outcome**

Have you ever, finally, after months of deliberation, started the first steps to something new when all you meet are **obstacles**, which get in the way of what you want to do. You might find people who won't co-operate or who aren't interested in you, or your project. There may be other things which block you, such as what you need not being available for weeks. It can all get rather frustrating. You might think these hurdles are about one thing, although they may turn out to be something quite different. Sometimes they indicate that you are doing things the wrong way, or maybe you should reconsider your strategy for achieving what you want. It's worth thinking about the different parts of making a change. It's often about approaching something from another point of view from how you normally deal with it. After all, if what you've been doing could have helped you change, you would have already done so. There is also the part of you which worries about where and when it will happen and how you might feel about that.

Think, too, about how you will be behaving in your new life. Can you imagine being the new person you want to become? You could begin to introduce a tiny bit of the new behaviour into your present situation so that you begin to make small changes. Then ask yourself if you have the required skills or whether you need some further training. Is what you want to do in line with your own values and outlook on life? How will the transformation you want affect your identity? How does it fit into your 'big picture', your life's purpose?

Going through these different parts of a decision may help you identify how to move forward, or where your block to progress might be, because until you try doing something new, how can you know whether it will work or not? You may feel it's rather like jumping off a cliff. You have to trust that there will be a soft landing.

However, when you finally make the decision to take action, you find many of the difficulties you worried about are only in your head and they fade away rapidly. A great shift in your thinking happens when you realise there are many different ways to achieve something. As a doctor, you may be used to following a standard routine when examining patients or solving problems. Changing your life may need a new approach. If you have come to this point in your life wanting to change, but wondering if you can, then it's important to recognise this. Notice how you approach a mundane task such as shopping. If you begin to understand the way you approach buying, then this may give you an insight into the way you undertake other things in life.

As with learning styles, people tend to have differing approaches to shopping. If you are strongly influenced by what an object looks like, you may not listen to what people tell you about the product or ignore any uneasy feeling about it, then you may find you can do things more effectively when you introduce these aspects into your decision making too. On the other hand, if you are not convinced about something and you predominantly hook into the visual aspects, you tend to make decisions based on the appearance of something, and you might realise that what's holding you back is the need to see more of what you are hoping to achieve. This could be pictures on paper or in your head.

Likewise you might be someone who connects when you just know, inside yourself, that it's right, it's the emotion you have about something. So, if the 'gut feeling' isn't there you may not want to proceed.

All this may be strange to you if you are someone who tends to have a way of doing something which you always follow. If what you want to do is to change and live a different sort of life then you need to explore new ways and be willing to encompass new ideas and ways of approaching them. As you begin to embrace a spirit of **openness**, you will allow diverse ways to do things to come into your mind. Listen to what others say, watch what they do, read more, think more and dream more. Notice how you feel as you do this and what gets you into a positive frame of mind.

Creating more space for fresh ideas can be physically as well as mentally rewarding. It's always beneficial to do some clutter clearing if you are stuck. It seems to be the physical movement, both of yourself and things which allows other shifts to happen too. It's quite remarkable what the effect of taking a few bags of clothes to a charity shop or clearing out a pile of old journals for recycling, has on you and your project.

Look out for **opportunities**. They are all around you but you will only be aware of them when you have the mind-set of authenticity, the real you. That's when others may call you 'lucky'. When you start to be open to possibilities you will find that there are more than you ever imagined. Just because you don't know of other alternatives right now, don't assume there aren't any. When your mind is open, things happen.

There is more than one way to go about what you want to achieve. Jot down, as a mind map, all your possible **options**, however unlikely some may be. Don't dismiss anything. Consider the pros and cons. You may be giving invalid reasons why you can't do something. Sometimes, opportunities aren't obvious until you decide to explore every possibility. You have to take a leap into the relatively unknown. Be brave. Take a risk.

Instead of thinking why you can't do something **original**, start to find ways you can. Don't make assumptions about what someone will say or how they might react to you. Mind reading has a habit of being incorrect. The only way you'll get a sense of what someone thinks is to ask them. You are not responsible for their reaction anyway. You will begin, instead, to decide on the **outcome** you want. Initially this is the goal which you have clearly defined and subdivided into small manageable steps. You've decided it is possible for you to achieve the goal so long as you put your mind to doing so. And you've set a date by when you plan to do it. You are all set for your journey of change. It might turn out to be as easy as ABC.

P is for

Passion	**Positive**
Passionate	**Posture**
People	**Power**
Persistence	**Purpose**

The driving force for change is **passion**, your passion. As the author of your own life you must feel the excitement of what you want so strongly that you know, with certainty, one way or another, you will get there. Unless you are **passionate** about what you want to do, you will find it difficult to maintain the momentum towards your goal especially in the face of opposition and discouragement from others.

If you find yourself on a lonely road, driven completely by your conviction you are on the right one, you may not want to involve anyone else. There is a fine line between doing something entirely on your own, because that's the only way you can get it done and finding someone to help in some way. It may be somebody to pick up the phone to, for a chat, or meet over a coffee, or it may be much more hands on assistance. However, those **people**, willing and able to support and motivate you to take the initial big step out of your comfort zone and start the process, are a valuable resource.

Whatever you decide to do will inevitably have an impact on someone else, too. So, being able to talk through the pros and cons, realise what might happen if you do, or if you don't do, what you propose, is all part of the process and can also be very useful. Become more aware of those able to offer encouragement and let go of those who try to discourage you.

Some of your supporters may be able to point out the good or bad aspects of your ideas, as they understand them. This can be very valuable. It's useful to have someone to discuss with you the things which might go wrong, so long as they are willing to enter into a dialogue, allowing you a chance to maintain equilibrium between your dreams and their practicality and how, therefore, you can take the ideas forward with a dose of realism thrown in. If you find several people who try to dissuade you from what you want to do, then you may need to step back from them and seek out someone who is on your side, if you are convinced about what you want to achieve. Sometimes it's tempting to give up after the first failure, especially when others say 'I told you it was a stupid idea'.

Don't give up when something doesn't work at first. Think of the way a baby learns to walk, falling over and getting up, over and over. You may have been rather shaky when you first put up a drip, wondering if you would ever be able to do it with ease, or you may have questioned if you'd ever know enough to pass an important professional examination. You may have failed and decided not to re-sit or, more likely, you may have recognised the importance of going back to the books and re-sitting, even if that meant several more attempts.

Persistence is a great asset which comes as a result of your passion, because you may be doing several things and yet not detect any noticeable result for a while. However when you keep going, or try again, perhaps with some slight difference because of what you learn, change will eventually occur. If no one seems to take any notice of you, repeat what you want them to hear. Keep repeating it. Say it in different ways, calmly, assertively, reasonably, and you will eventually succeed.

One of the most effective and important ways to bring about significant change in your life is to have a **positive** mental attitude. Notice how often you speak about, or hear something said, with a negative slant to it. You may set yourself up for a particular experience when you say things like, 'I'm dreading today', or 'This is going to be awful'. How much more likely you would be to have a positive experience if you changed those phrases to, 'I'm looking forward to today', and 'This is going to be interesting'. Instead of 'This is going to be difficult', say 'I can do it'. Be more aware when you listen too, the words you use; and also those used by others. You may be surprised at how many negative ideas are expressed in everyday conversation.

Language reflects your thoughts and emotions. When you change the words you use, there is a 'knock-on effect' on your thoughts and beliefs and on your actions. Your experience is likely to be related to your expectations.

You also need to change the way you move your body to change your life. This could be as simple as changing your **posture**, from round-shouldered and stooping, to a straight back and open chest, i.e. the body of someone ready for a new way of being. Can you feel depressed when you have a smile on your face and an open posture?

Trust yourself and understand that you have the **power** to make a difference to the way you live your life. Be confident that you will find the answer to what to do. When you have the courage to look for it, you will find what you seek. It is as likely to be inside of you, as outside. Notice how altering the way you interact with others and changing the way you behave, results in a reaction. Your life will change and possibly the others too, in response to what you do.

Whatever has happened in your life so far, you now have the choice to say or do something different.

The point of power is in the present moment.
Louise L Hay

From this very moment you can decide to live life differently. Even if what you do seems to have little external consequence; you will notice an internal result on your own thinking. When you think differently about a situation, your beliefs about yourself and your life's **purpose** change too. You begin to realise that what you want to achieve may be part of something referred to as 'the big picture' connected to what you want to leave behind you after you die. Your desired legacy may shape not only who you are as an individual but also who you are in the world.

But you have to start with first things first. Get the basics sorted. Clear out cupboards and sort out your environment. That's the basis from where your higher aspirations can grow.

Q is for

Quality	**Quest**
Quandary	**Question**
Quantity	**Quiet**
Queen	

Maybe a reason for delaying and not moving forward is to do with your ideas about standards, that is what is acceptable and what isn't. If you don't come up with something even better than everyone else, you get upset. If you want to give the best talk, or wear the most expensive clothes, then **quality** rather than tackiness might be important for you. However the expectation of perfection might be unrealistic and stop you from going ahead with the change you want.

Too many people, especially doctors, and perhaps you are one of them, use this as an endless excuse for procrastination. When you are about to do something you haven't done before you may want to be as good as possible. In the end, however, it's important to get started even if you doubt yourself. This may mean having someone to help and guide you just as you did when you learned various medical procedures. Were you perfect when you first put up a drip or did a lumbar puncture? Did the quality of your work improve as you reached the end of your house jobs compared with when you had just started? If you are sure that what you want to do is reasonable and potentially could be achieved by you then go for it and be prepared to learn and improve.

Be careful about setting yourself standards which you couldn't possibly ever achieve. This can lead to frustration and giving up completely. Instead, decide on small achievable goals, so that you can progress. Don't let your doubts overwhelm you. Just keep asking yourself, 'What will happen if I don't do this?', 'What will happen if I do?' and even, 'What won't happen if I don't do it?' and 'What won't happen if I do?'.

If you are in a **quandary** about how you could ever succeed remember that sometimes a silver standard is fine and acceptable. It's alright not to strive for gold every time. Be prepared to accomplish what you can in a reasonable time, then you can step it up as you achieve more. Don't let your dilemmas about success or the lack of it be all you think about.

Sometimes, it may be more important to go for **quantity**, when you are trying to achieve excellence. Get into the flow of what you are doing, such as writing up a backlog of medical reports, so that you can have a blitz on the work needing to be done and tackle as many reports as possible over a set period of time. Putting all your energy into a specific project and deciding to get it done can be very empowering and also prevents things becoming a drain on your enthusiasm. Make sure the result you want is what you are working towards, rather than what someone else wants for you.

If you are unable to make progress because of feeling intimidated, then imagine what it might be like to be a story book king or **queen**. Imagine walking into a situation confident, as if you rule the country, knowing you are right; you only have to give the word for your subjects to obey. When you next go into the situation you dread, be a king or queen. Your change in posture and emotion will affect the way you speak and the way you come across to others. You may be surprised by how the change in you has an effect on others too.

As a doctor you may be living mostly in your head, wanting to work out the logic, the reason for something, and what it all means. When you change the way you walk and move you will feel different and become more assertive, gradually getting used to the change.

Whatever your **quest**, whether it's to change your life completely or to improve the life you live already, don't forget to keep holding the vision of what you want in your mind's eye. Part of the process of change is realising that some of the going may be tough. There will be times when you wish you'd never started and want to turn the clock back. Once you've started, keep your focus on what it is you want to achieve.

Be prepared to change direction if necessary. You may not be able to go directly from A to B, there may be diversions on the way. Some of these might be worth exploring and may even lead you to a more interesting path to follow. You can check in from time to time and ask yourself whether what you want is still a reasonable and achievable goal or whether a new way is better.

If circumstances change, or maybe just as a result of working towards your goal, you may realise that what you have been striving for is not now what you want. That's alright, because it's what life is about – going with the flow, adapting, changing. It's not a rigid path. More often it meanders and changes in response to other things. When you meet opposition keep centred and don't allow yourself to be dragged into someone else's problem.

Don't just accept – ask, **question** and challenge your own and others' assumptions. Say 'no' when appropriate. You may stimulate your own thinking as well as the other person's thinking. This enables you both to have a useful and constructive discussion to better view how you each understand the situation. When you show empathy, the other person may become more aware of your point of view too, especially when you speak and move with confidence, as if you have the answer to everything.

At times, the whole world seems to be ganging up against you and your ideas and you begin to doubt everything. Find yourself a **quiet** place to sit and close your eyes and just breathe; let everything wash over you so that you can let it go; centre yourself and gather yourself together to move onwards with renewed determination.

R is for

Realist	**Relaxation**
Reality	**Request**
Recognise	**Resistance**
Reflect	**Results**

Some people might call you a pessimist although you say you are a **realist**, because you strongly believe nothing in your situation could possibly change, no matter what you say or do. You've 'been there and done that' so many times and all you ever get in response is resistance and resentment, so you don't believe one person can make a difference. Although you, along with others, talk with enthusiasm about how the situation could be improved, none of you do anything except continue to moan. It's frustrating when you know things could be better than they are and yet working out the steps to make it happen seems too big a task.

So nothing changes, even though the absolute very first step is what you may have been doing, admitting that something needs to change and exploring different options. Perhaps you don't do any of the things you thought of, because you are skilled at making excuses, such as 'If I do that, so and so will be offended or upset' or 'My colleagues don't want what I want, so I must be wrong'. You are expert too at reading people's minds and are sure you can foretell their reaction to what you might do. All these are ways in which you put off making changes to your life.

It often seems much easier to put up with that with which you are familiar, than to take the chance, not knowing for sure what the outcome will be. Getting out of your head into a place of trusting it will all work out for the best is a huge leap for you, but probably one which you will need to take sometime. It's scary though, even thinking about it.

To allay your fears it might be sensible to do a **reality** check. For example, 'Suppose it doesn't happen the way I want, what might be the consequences?'. Have you a plan B if plan A doesn't work out?

If your idea involves a drop in income, how much financial leeway do you have? If you don't have regular employment how would you pay the bills?[1] Ask yourself again these four questions.

- What will happen if I do this?
- What will happen if I don't do it?
- What won't happen if I do it?
- What won't happen if I don't do it?

You need to **recognise** and acknowledge your present situation without letting it stop you from making suitable changes.

It might be quite a juggling act to decide what you can drop from what you have been trying to keep in the air. If you are doing too much, or keeping too many options open your feeling of overwhelm may be severely reduced when you make some choices. Decide to explore one of your options fully. Give yourself the chance to consider what happens and then to make another choice to go on forward with it or to move on to another option. Instead of staying put doing something you don't want to do, discover what really fires you. And that's the way to go!

When you **reflect** on your life and what you want to achieve in the time you have left, you may suddenly realise that this is finite and undefined. It might be long or short. So why are you waiting to do what you really want to do? Why are you living a life along the lines of someone else's definition of success? Do you want the status of being at the top of your profession or do you want some precious time with your children while they are small? These are decisions only you can make but there will be pressure put on you from others to take one path and not another. Is it time to consider not only what you still want to accomplish but also what's important to you now?

When you think about the future, acknowledge what you have done up until now and recognise that you have gained many skills. You will be told if you don't do this and that now, that doors will close for you professionally. It's easy to get sucked into that argument for continuing to do a job you hate, instead of living a more balanced life. Be open to other definitions of success and trust that there will be new opportunities coming to you when you are open to them. So many doctors keep on their narrow treadmill of one job after another and forget that there is a world out there of non-medics, of satisfying jobs, of opportunities too, if you decide to look.

There are also some doctors who have grasped the meaning of work–life balance. Talk to them and notice what they do and don't do. They can teach you all you need to know to be a doctor *and* have a life. For instance, they will tell you to take some time out during each day to stop and reflect on what's happening. This could be a few seconds between patients to close your eyes and take a few deep breaths into your lower abdomen, or half-an-hour at lunch time not only to eat something but also to go for a short walk in the park.

A few minutes each day for **relaxation** is priceless for your health and wellbeing. When you take a few moments to check in with your body and scan through from your toes and legs, to your hands and arms, through your head and spine and abdomen and chest, it's a way to be aware of areas of tension to be removed by taking in a breath and as you breathe out to relax the tense area.

Often, the first step for changing your life for the better involves talking to the people involved and making a **request**. Be really clear what you want from them and by when. Don't expect them to be able to read your mind. It doesn't help anyone to complain without making what you want very specific. Ask, specifically, if they are prepared to do what you ask. It's easy to be frustrated by someone apparently not doing what you ask, but on reflection you may realise that you didn't tell them exactly what you wanted them to do and you didn't have their agreement to do it.

If you are still finding it difficult to get moving on the project, think about it more deeply. What is your **resistance** to making the changes you want really about? It may be fear, apprehension about change or of losing sleep if your solution doesn't work. Quite understandably you want to be absolutely sure before you make a move.

But can you ever be 100 per cent sure? Once you've checked out certain things then there will always come a point when you can't be sure. Life by its very nature is full of uncertainties. You can probably recall patients who recovered against the odds and others who died in spite of there being no obvious reason for this.

Let go of your wish to be perfect.[2] Instead, be prepared to take a chance and take that leap of faith towards what you really want instead of continuing as before. Are you letting the possible reaction to your ideas keep you in a situation which you don't like?

There has to come a time when you ask what's stopping you. You may find your excuses are wearing rather thin. Is your answer about your self-belief ('I'm not good enough', 'It wouldn't work for me'), or more about what others might think of you or your behaviour?

If you want the **results** you dream of, you have to take action. How about sooner rather than later? However much you talk about it, nothing changes until you do something. Nothing happens until you set the ball rolling. You have to do something, however small. You have to take the first step.

References

1 Harvey J (2004) I'm coming to the end of my registrar training. Should I do some locum work before I look for a practice? *BMJ Career Focus Advice Zone.* **328:** 92.

2 Kersley S (2003) Can you let go of being perfect? *BMJ Career Focus.* **327:** S76.

S is for

Sadness	**Success**
Seasons	**Support**
Self-care	**Synchronicity**
Self-esteem	**System**
Simple	

Perhaps you've actually started making changes and hoped to be happy at your accomplishments so far. You might, unexpectedly, find yourself not only beset with doubts, but also wonder why you feel some **sadness**, as though you were grieving. This tends to be part of the process because, just like mourning for the death of a loved one, letting go of the old to make room for the new is associated with feelings of loss. You might experience a gamut of emotions from sorrow to anger, from guilt to acceptance. Instead of being confused by this, expect it to occur

When you think again of the **seasons** of the year as a metaphor for what happens during life changes, you may understand more fully. Giving up the old life is like Autumn, a time for finishing, closing down, shedding the old. This is followed by Winter, when no growth seems apparent. It's bleak and bare on the surface until you realise that out of sight there are lots of things, dormant, waiting for the right time to germinate, preparing to emerge and burst forth in Spring, the time for new growth and new life. Then Summer comes when your new life is in full bloom.

The seasons of change are not necessarily the same as the current season of the year. You may even be going through more than one cycle of change and be in different seasons with each one.

Self-care is vitally important while all this is going on. If you neglect it you neglect your life. To be efficient and capable of initiating change you must look after yourself as well as you possibly can. When you look after your own needs as much as you look after those of others you become much better able to do your work.

What does self-care entail?[1] It means valuing and fulfilling yourself and your own needs; recognising you are important too, instead of only caring for others and fulfilling your role in relation to them. It's vital for your personal health and wellbeing to allot time and energy to yourself and your own needs.

If you find you are overwhelmed by tasks which others expect of you, so you have little energy left, then look at how well you prioritise how you deal with yourself. To look after yourself more effectively, start with noting what you plan in your diary. Recognise that this is as necessary as a meeting or a clinic. Make time for your own needs by managing your day more effectively.

By doing all this your **self-esteem** will be much, much improved too. When you feel good about yourself, you will be better able to be clear about what you want to achieve, when and how, with whom and where. You will be clearer about what is really important for you, your life purpose, your self-identity, whether your life is congruent with your values, and whether your needs are satisfied.

How can you align your values with how you live? The answer may be very **simple**. Ask yourself what is really important to you and what you need for a happy and balanced life. If your answer is that you need more time for yourself, your friends, your family, pursuing your own hobbies and also some time just to sit and connect with nature, then it may be as easy as saying 'no' to someone or something so that you can leave work at a reasonable time.

You have to decide to complete what has to be done for your patients, employer, and the Government during your normal working hours. It's as simple as making the decision not to do such and such any more. Decide how to deal with what would happen if you no longer take work home at the end of the day. If you don't take the briefcase, when will you do the work? You will find a way to be more efficient or more selective about what you do.

Just like many people, you probably either are, already, or want to be, successful. But have you ever stopped and asked yourself what **success** *really* means for you? Thinking about this might be useful to help you decide what to do. Is your definition of success imposed on you by others? Is it only in relation to work, or does it also include integrating all parts of your life so you are fulfilled, even after a busy day at work. Sometimes being a busy doctor can feel quite isolating. You see people going home at five o'clock and resent the work you still have to do. You hear your children saying that other people's mothers or fathers take them to this or to that and you wonder if you are missing their childhood years while you feed the ever hungry needs of your trust or deanery or the Government.

Everyone benefits from having **support** at times of change, even when you are just doing your day-to-day work. Do you have someone to talk things over with, who will listen and encourage you and also feedback what they hear you saying? It can be very useful to hear your ideas spoken as the other person hears them. Who or what supports you? Do you meet your colleagues occasionally to talk through some of these issues so that together you might be able to improve working practice for you all?

However, it's not all doom and gloom. When you step onto your new path you may be amazed how often **synchronicity** happens. You may be wondering how to do something and then you meet the person who knows the answer you are looking for! You may believe nothing can alter unless something is changed by those who control 'the **system**'. You may consider that you, as an individual, are powerless to have any influence. If that is what you think, then that will be your experience.

Big changes happen by someone doing something differently. This might involve asking a question, making a request, or giving an ultimatum. It could be you who makes the difference not only to your life but to others too. If one thing alters other things have to adjust too. Life is like a spreadsheet; when you change one thing, everything else changes too.

What could *you* do? What small step could *you* take towards living the life you want? Be proactive – don't wait for someone else. Talk about what you intend to do – don't make assumptions about the effect you will have on others.

Reference

1 Kersley S (2003) Looking after number one. *BMJ Career Focus.* **324:**S85.

T is for

Talk	**Time**
Tasks	**To-do list**
Technology	**Tolerations**
Think	**Trust the process**

If you know you want your life to be different and spend hours thinking about it, mulling over the pros and cons and wondering if there is more to think about, you could **talk** to as many people as possible, especially those who would be most affected and those who may have done something similar.

When you have a conversation, with an exchange of views, this is always a good way to check something out, when you want to make a change which may affect others as well as yourself. You might be surprised at their reaction. A good approach is to flatter them with how much you admire what they have achieved and then tell them about your vision. Tell them how you plan to work towards it. Be specific about what you want from them. This may be anything from 'Let me know your thoughts about this idea' to 'Please explain how to use this computer programme'. Remember to thank them again for listening and for any information and support they give you. Bear in mind that this is still your project and their opinions will be based on how they see the world, which is different from the way you do. So their comments are biased, whether they realise it or not, on how they would feel about doing this or that thing, or how your ideas might be different from how they imagined your life would be.

On the other hand, instead of being opposed to your idea they may be more supportive than you imagined and be prepared to encourage you to do your new **tasks**. They may not only give you their support, but also draw your attention to useful resources or share their experiences about something similar. Too often, making assumptions and worrying about what so and so might say if you do what you are thinking of doing, stops you from taking action. Yet you don't actually know for sure. You can't really read their mind.

Are you comfortable with using the Internet and computers? If not you may be missing out on valuable resources. What do you need to do to be more adept in this area? **Technology** is useful. You could become more efficient at managing your life by using your computer diary with reminders of engagements, for example. Use is not only for work and study commitments but you could also allocate personal time in your diary too. Appointments with yourself are as important as your other responsibilities. If you decide to do something (for example, swimming) it's easy to insert this into your electronic diary. In this way you can plan your day to include your self-care too.

When you are still wondering whether to do, or not do, what you want, **think** carefully about whether it's worth the emotional cost to you. Consider the effect your change may have on others and how their life might change too. Because, although it's important to value your own needs as a high priority, your change will affect those around you too.

You say you haven't time at the moment to do the things you dream of doing. It may be stating the obvious, but everyone has 24 hours each day. What varies is how you spend that **time**. Like it or not, if you want to do something extra you may have to stop doing something else. So this is a good time to reassess what you do, how you do it and whether someone else could do it. You might start by putting into practice whatever you've learned from courses or books about time management. These techniques will be useful and enable you to plan your day better and make good use of your time.

Be sensible about your **to-do** list. Plan to do what you can realistically complete each day and then do those things. Also become more adept at planning to do tasks over periods of time. If you want to complete something by the end of the month, work out what needs to be done by the end of the week, and week by week. This is a most important technique for getting things done.

There are also those things which you know you have to get around to doing some time or other known as **tolerations,** the irritating things you put up with, which you avoid doing – things like broken objects which need to be repaired or replaced, surfaces which need to be tidied, things to be taken for recycling and so on. You keep telling yourself that such and such needs to be done, or thrown away, or mended when you have the time, and that never happens. Complete all the tasks which get on your nerves without any further delay. They drain your energy so it's good to decide to do away with them once and for all.

Above all, develop a sense of confidence, an awareness of being able to **trust the process**, knowing that whatever happens is best for you at this time. Let go of your need to be certain, to be in control, to be too organised. There are times when these are useful attributes but when you are being led by your feelings and your vision for a better life, being too rigid may be a disadvantage. When considering doing something very different you need to tune into your body and your emotions as well as your logical mind. You need to recognise what makes your heart sing. And you won't feel that in your head! And if things go wrong, what then? There is always a lesson to be learned when things don't go right, as much as when things go the way you want. Ask yourself what went well, what you could do differently next time, and what you have learned. Next time you will benefit from these lessons and do things differently.

U is for

Undermine
Understand
Understatement
Unobtrusive

Unshakeable
Usual
Unusual

There's always someone, isn't there, someone who tries to **undermine** your enthusiasm. They tell you all the things which might go wrong with what you suggest and forget to tell you anything positive, even though, when questioned, they reluctantly agree you may have a few good points. Some people believe their role is to criticise everyone else and constant criticism can be daunting at times. If you switch your mind-set so that instead of being upset by this, you take the view that they may have a valid point or two. So, consider your response to their comments. Take a more positive stance and explain at least to yourself and to your critic, the advantages of doing what you plan. In fact, it's useful to do this anyway, to ask yourself what might go wrong, or what you would do if so and so happened. Instead of being put off by negative behaviour or comments, you could regard them as a useful resource to help you consider things which might go wrong.

Comments in relation to 'the sort of person you are' may help you to understand how others see you and how you would like to be seen by them. Become more of an observer not only of the way people behave but also of yourself. However, these sort of reactions from others can be hurtful and may be difficult for you. The thing to remember is that sometimes people react in a certain way because of their problems, or because they are envious of you and the actions you are taking. They may be angry at you for moving forward in an area in which they wish they had also been able to do so. Consider how different the person you would like to be is from the person you are, or are perceived to be. Sometimes doing this results in a shift in self-perception and a huge adjustment in inner awareness which results in a changed posture or expression and from that an alteration in the way your ideas are perceived by others. When you feel impatient about someone else's lack of understanding, or if they have their own agenda, take a moment to consider their point of view. Try to really **understand** where they might be 'coming from'.

Seek first to understand then be understood.[1]

Imagine if you were in their shoes, with their values. How differently would you view the world?

A common cause of misunderstanding or conflict is when the other person and yourself have a completely different motivation and desired outcome. You may discover this after some time when you thought you were both wanting the same thing. As you begin to understand why they are so resistant to you, avoid this happening by asking questions about their aims, find out more about their ideas, show interest, and congratulate them on what you appreciate about them. Then, when you have recognised better what drives them, you can tell them about your ideas. You may find they are more receptive to further discussion.

Don't be too quick to discourage another person and their ideas, without understanding their background. Even if you have to reject their proposal it helps both of you if this is done with respect, with an attempt to appreciate and encourage. You could say, 'That's an excellent idea and it's been useful to hear more about it', or 'I will certainly keep it in mind for the future. However, at this time with the budget we have, it won't be possible to implement it yet'.

How much better might you feel if this were said to you rather than, 'What a load of rubbish'! Too often doctors experience humiliation and feel undervalued. You could begin to change this culture by praising everyone who has completed something. All it takes is a simple 'well done'.

There seems to be, among doctors, a desire for **understatement**. However clever or brilliant you are, do you shy away from announcing your grand vision for the future, for fear of ridicule. This understatement of your aims and objectives or desired outcome, helps no one. Be bold and state what you want and explain your plan for achieving this.

Although your natural inclination might be to be **unobtrusive** at times when you are initiating change, it is better to be more forthcoming and clear about what you want. It might be to your advantage to be more assertive and state your intentions clearly.

You will be much more motivated when you are almost **unshakeable** in your enthusiasm and passion for your intentions. If they are things which will change your life you are the one to initiate the process. No one else is likely to feel as strongly about it as you. That's fine because everyone has a differing view of the world and yours is as valid as theirs. Your initial aim might be to change the **usual** routine, not only your own but also to involve others. Suppose you want to review the way you see patients in your clinic. Has anyone ever been logical about how to decide when to see the patient for a follow-up visit. Perhaps on the day you started the job you were shown the ropes by a colleague who told you to arrange follow-up appointments in three weeks. If you think your clinics are far too busy, then you could try bringing up the subject of follow-up appointments at your next meeting.

Even though the others may think your behaviour is somewhat **unusual**, especially if you've been thought of as a rather quiet retiring sort of person, this may make them sit up and take notice. Surely it's better than continuing as you've always done (because then you will get what you've always got)? So, keep your mind on your desired result and put all your energy into achieving this.

Reference

1 Covey S (1989) *The 7 Habits of Highly Effective People*. Simon and Schuster, London.

V is for

When you are more aware of your personal **values** you begin to understand why some things arise because of differing morals of the Government who set the targets, the managers who have to make sure they are achieved and the doctors who have to do the work to reach them. The surgery your patient needs may take too long so that you won't be on target for completing the required number of operations that week. Maybe you are working for, or with, someone who has very different standards, so that you find it difficult to get on with them. Values are the principles, the ethics, the ideals, by which you live. If you are unhappy, consider whether those of your employer are congruent with yours.

If you attach importance to spending time with each patient and are told you have a maximum of 10 minutes, your principles may be compromised and you feel stressed as a result. If you are someone who finds it difficult to say no, someone who won't consider going home until every possible task is done and more, then you need to ask whether you **value yourself**, and your own needs, enough.

This is all about work–life balance.[1] In order to have a balanced life you have to recognise that life is more than work, more than things you do for others; it's also about you and your needs. If you've been neglecting yourself, then start to do things you haven't done for ages and notice what a difference this makes to your life. Begin to give more priority to those things you used to love to do but since you became a doctor have neglected. If you used to play an instrument, get it out and play for 20 minutes. If you used to paint, designate some time for this. If you love to sing, find out where the local choir meets and join in once a week.

Talk to anyone who will listen to you about what you want to change. Don't just grouse about it, instead start to **verbalise**, to describe your dreams.

Tell your colleagues, your friends and your family what you would love to happen and how you intend to make the changes you want. Begin to talk as if it's possible, as if you are on your way to achieving it. Remember, however, that you already know, whether you are prepared to admit it or not, what has to be done and how to do it. You just need the motivation and encouragement to start. Don't say, 'I couldn't do that because I know what so and so will say ...'. Instead say, 'Yes that's fine. No problem'. You don't know until you speak to them. And when you do, always start by saying something complimentary. Follow this with the thing you want to ask (the 'meat') and then close the conversation by saying something nice again.[2]

The more you talk about how you would like it to be, and the more you explore ways that you could begin to make it happen, the more likely it is to become reality.[3] It's easy to be weighed down not only by the challenges at work but also by the demands and expectations of people at home. Consider how much of your daily routine at work or at home could be delegated. It's no help to say that no one else can do it as well as you. Maybe that's so, or maybe it's not. However you could teach the person to whom you delegate then allow them to do it. Perhaps some of what you do could be stopped altogether or done more efficiently. What will you do just for you, today, this week, this month?

How can you change things which seem to be overwhelming? You might start by having a **vision** of how life would be in your ideal world. See it, hear it, smell it, experience it, all while sitting in your own armchair. Do this regularly, every day for just a few minutes; it will have a huge effect.

Visualisation is the skill you need to do this. It is about picturing yourself in your perfect life in your mind's eye, on a regular basis. Start by thinking about what you want, imagine what your life might be like if it was going well. Find a quiet place, listen to some peaceful music and close your eyes. Take a few deep breaths, and starting with your feet be aware of the tension in your body, relaxing each area every time you breathe out. Imagine yourself in the life you wish for and notice with all your senses what is going on, how you are behaving, what you are saying, to whom you are relating. See yourself as though you are watching a video, or imagine stepping into the life you want. Not only watch, like watching a video or a film, but experience it too, by getting right into the picture so that you are there rather than being an onlooker, and you will see life going well for you.

Experiment with changing the scenario by making the colours brighter, the sounds louder and the feelings stronger. Decide which is best for you and enjoy being in that place. After a while open your eyes and, before you forget, write down what you thought about. You have the basis for working towards the life you imagined. Now you know how to **visualise** your ideal life, so practise this regularly. The more you experience what you want, in your mind's eye, the more likely it is that it will happen. It can take just a few seconds to replace a scenario you don't want with one you do. When you do this it is more likely to be what actually happens.

However, what you need more than anything is plenty of **vitality**. When you are passionate about achieving your goals you will have some already. But you also need to make sure you do what you can to improve and increase your vitality, by eating healthily, exercising regularly and generally looking after not only your body but your mind and spirit too. You need to be as fit as you can be when you begin your **voyage**, your journey to your new life. There may be rough seas ahead but also there will be calmness and wonderful experiences along the way to reaching your goal. Although it's good to have an eye on your destination remember to be in the present too and enjoy each day as fully as you can.

References

1 Kersley S (2001) Striking the balance. *BMJ Career Focus*. **323:** S2.

2 Kersley S (2002) Do your colleagues understand you? *BMJ Career Focus*. **324:** S117.

3 Kehoe J (2003) *Mind Power*. Zoetic, Vancouver, Canada.

W is for

Way forward	**Window of**
What	**opportunity**
When	**Win-win**
Why	**Wondering**

After all the discussion you want to find a **way forward**, and to do this you have to take a chance. You have to do something different and take some action. You have to be like the bird pushed out from its nest and trust that when you take a leap into the unknown, you will fly!

By now, hopefully, you will be clearer about your intentions and desired outcomes. You will have done a lot of thinking about **what** you want and how you can attain it. You will have defined this in terms of something specific so that you recognise when you have accomplished it.

When you get to the end of another busy day and sigh to yourself, 'I really need to get this work–life balance thing sorted', you are unlikely to make much difference to your life until you define this goal more precisely.

What does the term 'work–life balance' mean to you? It may mean something very different to your colleague. What it signifies to you might be spending time with your partner and family every evening; for someone else it may mean being able to swim 50 lengths of the pool on the way home. Work–life balance is likely to follow from finding the time and energy for different aspects of your life.

Medical work can dominate everything else if you allow it to. Be clear about this; you *are* entitled to a life too. You *can* find time to look after yourself, to spend time with your partner, friends, family and community. Spending all your waking hours either working or worrying about work is not a good balance. To make the changes you want, know your timescale and be clear by **when** you want your better life to become your new reality. People who do this are said to be more likely to attain their goals.

It is very important to set yourself a time limit for what you want to do and plan back from then. If you want to achieve something in six months decide what you have to do by the end of this month. You don't even have to be able to say **why** you want to reach your particular goal, although when people ask it may help to have some sort of reason to tell them which may or may not be your true motivation.

When you are really clear about what you want, by when, and how you can achieve it, you are better able to recognise any **window of opportunity** for taking the next step. People will say you have all the luck but it's more a matter of having your personal antennae switched on to pick up any possible leads to take your plans forward.

When you consider the pros and cons of what you want, you may believe that you can't let colleagues down, so may want to wait until this or that is in place. It's easy to make excuses for not starting. Some may be quite valid. If you only have another three months before you sit the examination, then you may argue that this would mean you have a recognised qualification. It might give you the reassurance that you could get another medical job if all your creative plans fall through. Having a plan B is a good idea, knowing that you can never be sure what you are going to do will work. Too many people use that doubt and don't ever dip their toe in the water of risk. Make sure these considerations have a time limit and be aware that there may never be an ideal moment.

If the whole idea of actually making changes is too scary, you may be using these reasons not just to delay but never to start at all.

Ideally, make your desired changes into a **win-win** situation for all the people affected. If you can, point out how others will benefit from what you propose and then you are more likely to get their co-operation to make it work for them as well as for you. A common experience is that others make changes when they see or experience you doing something different. So, not only do you change your own life but you may be enabling others to change theirs too. If you refuse to do the extra on-call sessions you are asked to do because you've decide your contracted on-call is enough you may be encouraging your colleagues to think about their on-call duties too. So they too may object and this may lead to more staff being appointed or a review of the system.

Do you spend too much time not doing anything because you want to make the right decision? Do you spend too long **wondering** whether to do this or to do that? You can deliberate for ever and nothing will change. You can spend an inordinate amount of time asking other people what they think. Yes it's good to talk, it's good to hear what they say, but in the end their life is not yours, their perspective is not yours.

The truth is that: you may or may not make the right decision. You will never know until you try. If it doesn't work the way you thought it would, then consider it as a learning experience to help you decide what you will do differently next time. The choice you have to make is about staying where you are (your comfort zone) even if it isn't what you want, or taking a big leap of faith into another place (your discomfort zone) with a chance, a possibility, that it may be a great improvement for you and your life. You may want to know what the practical 'back-up' is just in case what you do doesn't work out. You may want to ask yourself, 'What if ... happens?'. Ask yourself too, 'What will my life be like if I continue along the same path?'. If you imagine things getting worse, then doing nothing is not an option. You deserve better.

X is for

X	**X-ray**
X chromosome	**X-generation**
X-factor	**Xylophone**

There are some things in life which can have different interpretations, depending on where you are. For some doctors staying late every night and taking work home with them is about being an expert in their specialty or being completely prepared for the next examination. For others, it is an incursion into their private lives and upsets the work–life balance they strive for.

Like life, the letter **X** is multi-meaning. It's a symbol which touches many things, from 'You are wrong' to 'a kiss'. Your mood may change from distress or sadness if your work is covered with lots of Xs or to elation and happiness when the same symbols are at the end of a letter or email.

When written as Roman numerals it represents time as 10 o'clock or 10 years as part of a date. It signifies the passage of time, and the certainty that we only have this life and that the minutes and years tick by relentlessly. You may be aware of this especially on New Year's Eve when you realise another year has passed and nothing much has changed since the last lot of resolutions. On important documents X points to the place to sign your name, or to fill in your answer (X marks the spot).

How you interpret what X means depends on the context. Like many things in life, circumstances are important. You might be sure something has a certain explanation but when you think about it from another perspective, there may be a completely different interpretation.

If you want to change your life, others may not see the situation you are unhappy with in the same way you do. It's useful to hear how they understand the situation because this may either strengthen your determination to do something about it or give you a better understanding and so help you cope.

A useful habit to acquire when considering change which may involve you making requests of others is telling people what they do right (a metaphorical kiss?), before you tell them what they did wrong, Then they are more likely to be receptive to hearing you. It's all part of good communication.

You have at least one **X chromosome** as part of your genetic make-up. However, over half the population have two! There are more women becoming doctors nowadays in the UK so there is an ongoing adjustment in the medical profession's culture to be more in touch with the needs of women in relation to being mothers. There is also an acknowledgement that everyone, male or female, is entitled to work less than full time if they wish, and has the choice to enjoy time away from work, to be part of their family and their community.

You have needs for rest and relaxation and are entitled to an opportunity for these, whether you have one, two, or more X chromosomes. Coping with a busy medical or other professional job in addition to a young family is something many doctors have to do even though they find it difficult juggling so many balls in the air. If you do this well you may be a person who has the **X-factor**, that indefinable something which enables you to seemingly do the impossible.

However, if you aren't coping and find it difficult, you can challenge the system by making changes yourself. Part of positive communication is about recognising that there is more to everyone than the person you see in front of you. Unfortunately, it's easy to make unconscious judgements about people based on their appearance or body language.

Imagine there was a special sort of **X-ray** to enable you to understand the internal world of a person. This could prevent you from making lots of assumptions about that individual based on your own background and culture. Since you cannot access the internal world in this way, be very clear in your conversations what you are asking. Be specific about the details and the time by when you want something done. Be aware that not only the words of your conversation but also your body language and your own emotions affect communication. Most of all listen to the answer the other person gives you. Have they agreed or not? If they haven't actually agreed to your request, don't make assumptions, because then your expectations won't be fulfilled. They may have decided not to do what you asked because they don't want to, or don't feel capable of doing it or can't understand the reason for the request. Their values may be different from yours.

Perhaps you were born between the mid-60s and the mid-70s, and are part of what is known as **generation X**.[1] If you are in this age group you may not be prepared to put up with the different work ethics of older people. You may be determined to have more time for yourself and your family. You may want to travel and work intermittently. In order to have this sort of life you like the idea of more flexible working conditions or starting your own business. Doctors, for example, might decide to be an associate general practitioner,[2] rather than a full-time partner. Older doctors may find it difficult to understand the ethos of younger doctors who want to do more than spend most of their time working.[3] They may also be rather envious of these doctors who say enough is enough, when they look back and realise they just accepted their life as a doctor to be all-encompassing. These are two extremes. Can you choose a middle way to be a professional and have a life too?

If you've enjoyed and now neglect your creativity, what's stopping you from reintroducing it into your life on a regular basis? What would you like to bring back into your life? What would reconnect you with the creative side of yourself again? Whether it is learning about Art History or playing the **xylophone** or whatever is your favourite instrument, doesn't really matter. It's about spending some time each week absorbed in something you love to do. Can you commit to spending say half-an-hour a couple of times a week doing that? When you do you may find yourself on the path to your new life.

References

1 Coupland D (1992) *Generation X*. St Martins Press, New York.

2 Marshall L (1997) Associate General Practitioners. *BMJ Career Focus*. **315**: S2.

3 Adams D (2004) Generation gripe: Young doctors less dedicated, hardworking? *AMN News*. **2 February**.

Y is for

Yardstick	**Yesterday**
Year	**Yoga**
Yearn	**Yourself**
Yes	

Have you ever felt frustrated by the feeling that this life isn't really what you dreamed it would be like when you set out as a medical student? There is a common misconception among doctors which is that you have to work exceptionally hard foregoing everything else, just for a while, just until you pass that examination or get onto the next rotation, or become a consultant, and then miraculously everything will be alright.

However, what you may discover is that each level of the hierarchy brings its own frustrations and challenges so that you find yourself craving for the next step up. The idyllic job never seems to happen; you get more and more overwhelmed with the amount of work to fit into a day and the responsibility of it all.

Perhaps your **yardstick** for accomplishment comes from another generation. Is it time to invent your own measure of success which isn't based on the amount of time spent in the ward or the surgery? You can define, for yourself, what having a life means to you. If you are told not to do this or that, ask yourself whether the other person is coming from a place of their own personal regret for their own wasted life, or whether they wish they had the courage you demonstrate to question the system.

Look ahead a **year** from now and imagine what would you like to be doing. Imagine what might be better and what might be worse or not have changed. Where will you be, with whom and is your imagined life better than the one you are in now?

You may **yearn** for a better life as much as you want but unless you take some action you will still be unsatisfied in another 12 months. Because, as you know, you can think about things forever and nothing actually changes until you do something differently. And when you do that, shifting something, even if it seems unrelated to what you want, the energy changes and you may find other things start to change too.

There is plenty written about saying 'no' in personal development books and articles. It's a useful word to use more frequently. However **'yes'** is a word to think about too. It has the power to change your life, when used appropriately. When you say it in relation to change, things start to happen.

Remember to say 'yes' to time for rest and relaxation, for fresh air during the day and healthy food at lunch time. It means saying 'yes' to leaving your workplace to go home at a reasonable time, finding time to look after your body, mind and spirit.

You may find you are saying 'no' more often than you used to. When you say 'no' what are you also saying 'yes' to? Opportunities may present themselves to you. Don't ignore them. Say 'yes'. If your gut instinct says go for it, then listen and act accordingly, if you are brave enough!

Many people spend a huge amount of energy and time going over and over something in the past which can't be changed. You may view the world differently as a result of what happened. If this memory is overpowering and you really can't get rid of a distressing story then talking to a counsellor or an NLP (neuro-linguistic programming) practitioner may be useful.

On the other hand, if you can, remind yourself that **yesterday** has gone and things happened which can't be changed. Think about how your past has impinged on your actions in the present and decide to look forward rather than back, towards the future, with all its new possibilities, rather than the past. Be engaged in the present.

One of the things which may help you make the transformation is movement. This doesn't necessarily mean going to a gym or running, but it could be something more gentle such as **yoga**, which helps you connect again with your breath, be more centred, and relax after a hectic day. As you learn to integrate your movements with your breath you become more flexible, not only in your body, but in your mind too.

Making big changes in life can be very stressful, so it's important not to neglect **yourself** during the change. If you begin to feel overwhelmed by all the things you have to do when circumstances are new, you may not feel as confident as usual. What can you do?[1] You can put yourself first, be present now and think about your future. Be creative, and explore every possibility to enable you to find the way for you to move forward and transform your way of being.

There may be other ways to have a fulfilling life as a doctor, or by using some of the skills you have from training as a doctor and then ways to progress become clearer. When you are clear not only in the goals you set but also who you are as a person and what is most important for you, now, in this life of yours, then you are likely to make what you want happen. And when you do that other parts of your life change too.

Reference

1 Kersley S (2002) Looking after number one. *BMJ Career Focus.* **326:** S109.

Z is for

Zap	**Zest**
Zeal	**Zigzag**
Zenith	**Zoom**
Zero hour	**Zzz . . .**

When you are working in a very busy job it's easy to be swept along by it with hardly any time to take a moment to design your very own strategy for change. Whatever happens, don't let your day-to-day activities **zap** your energy so that at the end of the day you are unable to do the things you want. If you plan mini-breaks during the day this will help you feel better anyway and give you some space to consider different options. These breaks could be very short, even a minute of centring and taking a deep breath into your lower abdomen, and as you breathe out being aware of and letting go of any tension in your shoulders, your neck and anywhere else.

Since it's so easy to be swept along by the demands of the job it's important to remind yourself why you want to do what you want to do in order to keep your **zeal**, your enthusiasm and passion alive for your desired outcome. Believe in yourself and what you want for your life so single-mindedly that not only might you persuade others, but also, your enthusiasm will encourage them to support you. When you do this you will move towards your desired life and reach the **zenith**, the fulfilment of what you aim for. It is within reach and is worth all your efforts.

There will be times during the process of change when you are aware of a **zero hour**, the epiphany of all your efforts, the moment when you have to jump into the unknown. You will know it, perhaps because you have a strong emotion, 'This is it, the chance to do it,' or may have someone who seems to call you to where they are, 'Come on in the water's lovely!' they seem to say, 'Look I did it. You can too'. At that moment the world may seem to stop still for a moment, waiting for you to say 'Yes, here I come' and to jump in with

zest, or to let the gremlins decide your life again as you back away and say 'Not today thank-you'.

If you really want to live instead of just existing, then decide to listen to your heart, see the possibilities and get off that treadmill. Instead of work, work, work and little else except for sleeping and eating, you could enjoy life to the full once more. However, expect to take a **zigzag** path to get to that place. For every few steps forward you may also take several backwards.

It's a common experience that you make massive changes and then reach a plateau. Some people give up at this stage and believe they have failed. It's important to hang on and keep your goal in mind, because after a while you'll make more progress. All of a sudden you may realise you are almost there. All you have to do then is to **zoom** in and claim your prize, the prize of having the life *you* want which encompasses everything that is important to you – a life in which you've set the parameters for success, in which you have time for satisfaction working as a doctor, and as a parent, a son or daughter, a brother or sister, a part of a larger family, a part of a wider community, and a part of the world.

If you've developed a habit of noting what's happening in your life in a journal each day then you will have a good way to reflect on this process of change. Reflective writing is a powerful way to monitor what's going on for you.[1] Remind yourself regularly of your goal, what it is you really want at this time of your life. Be prepared to change this if you discover something else more appropriate, because it's only when you start along the path that you will know if it's the right path or not.

If your goal is to make a major change, such as changing specialty or even leaving medicine completely, don't beat yourself up about wishing you'd known better and chosen more appropriately in the past. Rather, put it down to life's rich experiences and in the knowledge that no knowledge is wasted; each experience helps to form you into the person you have become and will be in the future. So, as you continue on your journey through life, set yourself tasks to complete each week to move you towards it bit by bit.

But remember, always remember, to have enough sleep (**Zzz** ...!) If you want your dreams to come true you have to first allow yourself the time and permission to dream (asleep or awake). When your disturbed nights on-call leave you sleep-deprived, you can't go about your day-to-day activities as efficiently as usual. To counteract this, you could try having 'power naps' during the day to boost your energy. Or make sure you have extra sleep with a few early nights. To have enough oomph to make the changes, you need not only enough sleep but also an awareness of your best time of the day when you have most get-up-and-go. Adequate sleep is vital not only for your health and wellbeing but also for coping with change.

Reference

1 Bolton G (2001) *Reflective Practice, Writing and Professional Development.* Paul Chapman Publishing, London.

Why an ABC of Change for Doctors?

You've reached the end of the alphabet for change. Which letter pushes your buttons? What words are relevant for *your* process of change?

Asking questions of yourself and others is just the beginning. By challenging yourself and the system you may discover that more change is possible than you ever previously imagined. When you initiate tiny changes they spread, like ripples after even a small pebble is dropped into a pond.

> *If you don't ask the right questions, you don't get the right answers. A question asked in the right way often points to its own answer. Asking questions is the ABC of diagnosis. Only the inquiring mind solves problems.*
>
> Edward Hodnett

You've read the book. You've noticed thoughts flitting through your mind in relation to your situation and now the challenge is: What next? Put the book back on a shelf and forget about it all? Or decide to give it a go and open doors to something exciting and different? It's your choice.

You could:

- *Carry on as usual.* Put your desire for change to the back of your mind once more. If you do this you might find thoughts which surface from time to time, and you sigh and say, 'If only I'd done something about the situation, years ago'.
- *Recognise how change involves doing something a little out of the ordinary.* After considering various options, you decide how and when to plan and develop a strategy to implement what you want to do.
- *Acknowledge that now is the time for you to change.*
- *Take the first step, however uncertain.* This will begin to lead you to where you want to go.

There is no guarantee your journey to change your life will be an easy and straightforward one. It may twist and turn presenting you with obstacles to be overcome along the way. At every point you may be confronted by decisions about whether to go on or to stop.

Does that mean you should stay where you are? That depends on you and the choices you make. Sometimes it seems much easier to stay where you are.

If you want to change your life, take the uncertain road to your dream.

Even though you will find yourself asking ...

- Am I on the right path?
- Shall I continue or go back?
- What do I really want?
- Should I do what I want or what someone else wants me to do?

... Bear in mind whose life you are living and be clear about what you want and why. Keep focused on your purpose and ride the storm.

As a result of the integration of your past experiences and your present reality, it will all come together with meaning. The journey may take years to get to this stage or it may be a very short journey. Since the only certainty in life is change, there is always another call to another journey and for each one there is the question, 'Shall I answer this call or not?'.

Where are you on your journey of change? Whether you are just starting a new one or completing one you've been on for sometime, don't give up. Keep going. You *will* get there if you really want to and you recognise how great life could be compared with the way things are now. You will also realise that there are some very good and positive things about your present life which perhaps you weren't able to appreciate before, because going on a 'hero's journey'[1] helps to give you great insight into the good things about what you have now. Perhaps also wonder why it took you so long to discover that life now isn't as bad as you thought it was.

Any change can be stressful. It may involve you going through the grieving process for what you are leaving in order to achieve what you want. So be prepared for moments of doubt, guilt, sadness and anger. It's all part of the course until you reach acceptance of your new and changed situation. It takes time for this to become part of you and you part of it.

Ask yourself this question now, 'Am I living the sort of life I really want?'. If the answer is 'Yes', that is fantastic. Well done! If the answer is 'No', the next questions are: 'What do I want in my life which isn't there now?' and 'What is the first step to make this happen?'.

Don't delay any more. Change your thinking and your behaviour will change too. From this moment your life can change for the better.

In a nutshell, all you have to do to change your life is to be clear what you want and what you don't want. Change is simply a matter of going from A to Z, one letter at a time.

Just do it.
Nike advertisement

In these matters the only certainty is that nothing is certain.
Pliny the Elder

They always say time changes things, but you actually have to change them yourself.
Andy Warhol

Reference

1 Campbell J (2003) *The Hero's Journey: Joseph Campbell on his life and work.* New World Library, Novato, CA.

Further reading

Bolles R (2003) *What Color is your Parachute?* Ten Speed Press, Berkeley, CA.

Buzan T (2004) *Mind Maps at Work: How to Be the Best at Work* Harper Collins, London.

Campbell J (2003) *The Hero's Journey: Joseph Campbell on his life and work.* New World Library, Novato, CA.

Covey S (2005) *The Seven Habits of Highly Effective People*, Simon and Schuster, London.

Dalai Lama and Cutler H (1999) *The Art of Happiness: A handbook for living.* Hodder & Stoughton, London.

Forster M (2000) *Get Everything Done.* Hodder & Stoughton, London.

Gerber M (1995) *The e-myth Revisited.* Harper Business, New York.

Kline N (1999) *Time to Think.* Ward Lock, London.

McDermott I and Jago W (2002) *The NLP Coach.* Piatkus Books, London.

The Newfield Network www.newfieldnetwork.com

Pearson C (1991) *Awakening the Heroes Within.* Harper, San Francisco.

Richardson C (1998) *Take Time for Your Life.* Broadway Books, New York.

Robbins A (2001) *Unlimited Power.* Pocket Books, London.

Index